Clarity

Crack the Code to Healing Body, Mind, and Emotions from the Inside Out

by
Nikki Engels

Contributing Authors:
Devi S. Nambudripad, M.D., D.C., L.Ac., Ph.D. (Acu.)
Benjamin K. Redman, O.D.
Vijai Khan, D.C.
Sloane Ketcham

Clarity Publishing House, Inc.

Copyright © 2019 by **Clarity Publishing House, Inc.**

ISBN-13: 978-0-578-59802-4

Clarity: *Crack the Code to Healing Body, Mind, and Emotions from the Inside Out.*

All rights reserved. No part of this publication may be reproduced, distributed or transmitted in any form or by any means, including photocopying, recording, or other electronic or mechanical methods, without the prior written permission of the publisher, except in the case of brief quotations embodied in critical reviews and certain other noncommercial uses permitted by copyright law.

Although the author and publisher have made every effort to ensure that the information in this book was correct at press time, the author and publisher do not assume and hereby disclaim any liability to any party for any loss, damage, or disruption caused by errors or omissions, whether such errors or omissions result from negligence, accident, or any other cause.

Adherence to all applicable laws and regulations, including international, federal, state and local governing professional licensing, business practices, advertising, and all other aspects of doing business in the US, Canada or any other jurisdiction is the sole responsibility of the reader and consumer.

Neither the author nor the publisher assumes any responsibility or liability whatsoever on behalf of the consumer or reader of this material. Any per-ceived slight of any individual or organization is purely unintentional.

The resources in this book are provided for informational purposes only and should not be used to replace the specialized training and professional judgment of a health care or mental health care professional.

Neither the author nor the publisher can be held responsible for the use of the information provided within this book. Please always consult a trained professional before making any decision regarding treatment of yourself or others.

Cover Designer: Danijela Mijailovic

Editor: Wayne H. Purdin

Free Gift

Thank you for taking the time to check out this book! I've created a special downloadable workbook for you to use as you work through the content of this book. Feel free to visit www.nikkiengels.com/downloads and opt in for a printable download of the workbook.

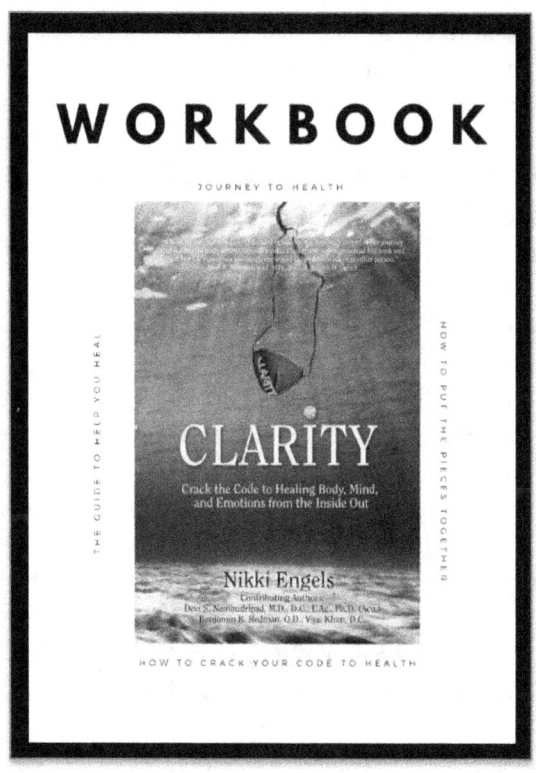

Testimonials

My hope is to allow you to find more credibility in my journey with these doctors' and authors' words, so that you can confidently start your own journey.

Words From Benjamin K. Redman O.D.

I remember that first visit with Nikki very clearly. I have known Nikki since we were kids and it's also not often a young healthy patient has sudden vision loss. It's never the same when it's a person you know, and this was definitely one of these rare unfamiliar situations with someone very familiar. As an eye doctor, there are a series of words and diagrams that become very fluid to explain different eye diseases and reassure the patient; none of that would help this time. In fact, until further testing was done, I wasn't sure what type of path this eye condition would take Nikki down, but I should have realized Nikki would rather make a path than follow. Now, I hope she will lead others with eye conditions to follow her example in taking control and making their own amazing paths, just like Nikki did.

"The eyes are a window into the soul." I have told many patients this phrase. From a medical perspective I usually discuss how the back of the eye is the only place we can see blood vessels not covered by skin. This is very important, especially in diabetic patients because it does represent all the small vessels we cannot see all the way down to the feet. After working with Nikki, I have changed my view of this phrase from a simple medical explanation. In the back of Nikki's eye there was a challenge, and it ended up being a very clear window into her soul.

Words From Dr. Vijai Khan

When I first met Nikki, she presented to my office with many concerns and questions about the condition of her eye and whether or not I would be able to help her with her condition. She also had many other symptoms to discuss, but was mainly concerned about her eye. I explained that for each person different allergens can affect different parts and tissues of the body in different ways. I tried to explain how, through NAET, we can energetically make those substances agree with the body as they should. She seemed very open to this idea and wanted to proceed with testing the various foods, chemicals, environmental allergens, and emotions. As we began muscle response testing, it became apparent that there were a multitude of various foods, chemicals, and emotions that were causing different symptoms and even affecting the eye.

As we began to work through a number of foods, some of the physical symptoms of aches and pains and digestive problems subsided. As we went through more chemical and environmental allergens, even more of the symptoms subsided. Week by week and month by month, Nikki slowly improved. As she continued with care from her optometrist and ophthalmologist, she would continually get scans of the part of her eye in question. I enjoyed watching her excitement as she would bring back each scan with improvement. There were a number of emotionally traumatic events from her life that also played a role in her health. As we connected how the emotions from some of these events played a role in her health, she slowly realized the importance of taking time to address her emotional health and trying to increase positive energy into her life.

The journey to health was by no means easy for Nikki. She has developed into such a positive person, and people are drawn to her positive energy. She has a wealth of knowledge, not only from a Yoga instructor and fitness instructor standpoint, but she possesses a great knowledge of how to help others have a positive attitude, even when negative life events occur. It has been a complete joy to watch Nikki improve from the first time she presented in our office with so many health problems to where she has improved today, not only with her eye, but with the other symptoms and emotional challenges she's overcome.

Words From Author Sloane Ketcham

Nikki's book takes you through her incredible true story of personal healing, overcoming what seems to be impossible at every turn. She recounts each moment with love and hope, giving the reader raw, behind-the-scenes, practical approaches to alternative healing methods that actually work. Nikki's triumphs prove that we all have everything we need to heal from within.

As a Kanaka (native Hawaiian), I grew up knowing that Hawaii is a special place. The islands are full of mana (power). Some say this mana comes from our ancestors; they say the islands are a spiritual vortex, forged together and brought to life by mother earth and father sky. Nikki's story is a compelling example of the magic Hawaii holds for anyone who hears its call.

The truth is, not everyone who comes to Hawaii feels this connection, and not everyone can feel its mana. Hawaii calls to its sons and daughters all across the world, regardless of race, color, or creed. The only thing necessary to receive its love is to be willing and open, like Nikki.

When I was sick as a kid, no matter what the ailment, my grandfather's remedy was always the ocean. He taught me to use the ocean for play and relaxation, but, most importantly, to turn to it for healing and sustenance. As native people of this land, we've been taught to respect and appreciate all that nature provides. Our state creed is *Ua Mau ke Ea o ka 'Āina i ka Pono*, which translates to "The sovereignty/life of the land is perpetuated in righteousness." That is to say, Hawaiian soil is holy, it's sacred, it's one of a kind, it's living and breathing, and here to serve its people but expects in return love and appreciation.

Nikki's story of healing is a testament of what Hawaii has to offer, beyond the beautiful beaches and pristine countryside, it's the living example of love, in Hawaiian, we call this aloha!

Dedication

This book is dedicated to my amazing husband, children, sisters, mother-in-law, and friends who have helped me stay strong and fight for what I knew in my heart was possible in this healing journey.

Words from my husband:
You're a force of good, a beautiful healing power in this world. Your words are helping people have the confidence to go and heal themselves through understanding the problem at a deeper level. –
I love you - Gary

Table of Contents

Foreword by Dr. Devi S. Nambudripad x
Part 1 1
   Introduction 1
   Chapter 1: The Beginning of My Story 2
Part 2 35
   Chapter 2: Saying "Enough" 36
      What You Can Do: Steps 1-4 39
   Chapter 3: Connecting the Dots 43
      What You Can Do: Steps 5-8 46
   Chapter 4: Gut Health 53
      What You Can Do: Steps 9-12 60
   Chapter 5: Cutting the Stress 64
      What You Can Do: Steps 13-16 74
   Chapter 6: Finding Outside Help 77
      What You Can Do: Steps 17-20 90
   Chapter 7- Believe 95
      What You Can Do: Steps 21-24 105
   Chapter 8: Love and Yoga 111
      What You Can Do: Steps 25-28 123
   Chapter 9: Taking My Life Back With NAET 128
      What You Can Do: Step 29 135
   Chapter 10 -Make Growing Your Goal 138
      What You Can Do: Step 30 139
   Resources Page 140
   About the Author 141

Foreword
by Dr. Devi S. Nambudripad

I consider writing forewords for authors who share my interest and vision as an honor. But when the author is also a patient who embraced NAET and achieved true health through the treatments, it is an inspiration!

I was first introduced to Nikki Engels through her warm introductory letter that I received on September 8, 2019. In her letter she gave an overview of her complete recovery from her rare genetically oriented eye disorder, and she detailed the restoration of her vision with the help of NAET treatments from a local NAET practitioner. She also shared her decision to write a step-by-step informational book to reach out to other patients with rare eye diseases. Nikki was hoping that if she shared her cumbersome journey, through various avenues and solutions for her diagnosed genetic eye disease, this would encourage others with similar problems to find a NAET practitioner who could help them solve their mysterious medical issues.

I liked her openness. I was also impressed by her generosity and willingness to share her NAET success story with others who suffered from similar health problems, now living in fear without finding a sensible solution. Even if just one person read her book and took her life experience seriously, she would help save the life of another person.

If she was successful in promoting her book, then many people would also live normally again. According to current statistics, 11 million people suffer from macular degeneration globally. I happily agreed to write the foreword knowing the potential power of this story by Nikki.

In her book, Nikki shares the unimaginable amount of physical, physiological, and emotional trauma and stress that she endured in her life before she received a proper diagnosis for her condition. The prognosis that came with her diagnosis was shocking to her initially. That didn't stop her. Once she gathered her composure, this brave woman set out on her journey in search of a permanent solution to restore her vision.

A born researcher, she decided to maintain a thorough record of her journey that led her through several difficult roads. This involved ongoing therapies, supplements, medicine, different doctors or therapists, and protocols that helped her or made her worse during this long journey prior to finally receiving a proper diagnosis from a renowned ophthalmologist.

The diagnosis of genetically oriented advanced myopic degeneration and neovascular membranes sent chills through her spine and fears through her heart, especially when she was told there was no cure for this disorder. The only way known to keep this under control was through repeated injections of medicine into the eye at regular intervals for the rest of her life!

This determined woman decided to continue her search to find a solution for her unique diagnosis. Soon, she found a NAET practitioner, Dr. Vijai Khan, who believed that the cause of most human health problems including eye disease was rooted in some form of undiagnosed allergy. He informed her that the allergy could be from food, chemical, environmental factors, or a result of accumulated, unresolved emotional traumas since childhood. He said it may take many office visits to resolve the problem through NAET. But he was willing to work with her in order to see if she could restore her vision permanently through NAET treatments.

She was thrilled to hear this news that someday, after she had eliminated these allergies, she might have an opportunity to restore her vision. She began NAET right away and continued to receive NAET treatments three times a week to eliminate her genetically oriented food, chemical, and environmental allergies. The NAET practitioner also helped her to eliminate the effect of numerous emotional traumas she had accumulated since childhood, since they were also contributing to her ill-health.

She continued to receive injections in her eye as needed from her eye specialist along with NAET treatments until she received the final diagnosis and confirmation from her eye doctor of the complete cure of her condition. That was also demonstrated in the optical coherence tomography (OCT) scans. To her, the diagnosis of a rare genetic eye disease is history now. The step-by-step record and presentation of her treatment approach along with all reports of her monthly OCT scans from her ophthalmologist is presented in this book in chronological order from the beginning. This story is well explained and convincing. I am sure once you read her adventure, you will agree.

Nikki has done a great job explaining what NAET® is all about, but I want to give you a quick introduction to help you understand her story better. Nambudripad's Allergy Elimination Techniques, known as NAET, is a non-invasive, drug free, natural, holistic solution to eliminate allergies of all types and intensities, from mild to severe sensitivity, including anaphylactic reactions. NAET uses a blend of selective testing and treatment procedures from acupuncture/acupressure, allopathic, chiropractic, nutritional, and kinesiological disciplines to balance the body bioenergetically so that it can get beyond any intolerance to the electromagnetic energies found in its living environment.

NAET was developed by me to overcome my genetically originated allergies and acquired sensitivities from exposure to pesticides since childhood that led to ongoing allergies and sensitivities through childhood and early adulthood until I discovered NAET. Within a few months of my discovery, I eliminated most of my allergies. Since 1983, I have been treating patients with this technique. Since 1989, I have also been teaching other health professionals how to administer NAET treatments. Since 2016, NAET has been taught through online seminars. Dr. Khan was taught through this current format, and we are finding that students learn the technique better when it is at their own pace. To date, more than 10,000 licensed practitioners have been trained in NAET procedures and are practicing all over the world. For more information on NAET training or for a NAET practitioner near you, log in to NAET website: www.naet.com.

According to NAET experience and theory, hidden sensitivities and allergies are the cause of numerous health problems. Often, some emotional events happened to the individual in this lifetime or the emotional traumas happened to their ancestors before they were born and carried to the individual through DNA or genetic transfer. This led to energy blockages in various parts of the body, thus causing hidden sensitivities, allergies, and allergy-related health disorders, including vision loss. You may read the books, *Resetting Your Emotions,* and *Say Goodbye to Illness* by Devi S. Nambudripad, available from www.naet.com or amazon.com bookstores to learn more about emotional events triggering unsolved health problems.

For those whose lives are merely disrupted by the discomfort of allergies or sensitivities, allopathic allergy treatments with simple antihistamine or topical remedies can bring some relief. But for more serious sufferers, long-term complete avoidance is the only solution traditional allopathic medicine can offer. Most people are not determined like Nikki; instead, they resort to a lifetime of depriving themselves of the many things in life that would otherwise bring them joy and fulfillment. Even with avoidance, there is no guarantee that hypersensitive persons will be able to stay away from every situation and still remain reaction free. Once symptoms become chronic, they respond poorly and possibly not at all to other treatments. Allergic symptoms may initially begin in one area of the body and eventually may involve various organs, giving rise to multiple organ symptoms, such as arthritis, asthma, or autoimmune disorders or other commonly seen health problems.

Often, the immediate trigger may be the chemical contaminants of items used daily. After over 36 years of allergy practice, I have learned that almost any symptom can be the result of an allergic reaction. When the allergies are detected and identified using NAET testing techniques, patients have two choices: (1) Complete avoidance or (2) Elimination of the allergic reaction by desensitizing for the allergen via NAET. In most cases, allergy elimination to the desensitized allergen through NAET is permanent.

Using NAET methods, one can re-program the brain, body, and their interactions with previously exposed unsuitable energies to harmless energies that might even help maintain a better immune system with later exposures after completion of NAET treatments.

Stay in health,
Dr. Devi S. Nambudripad, MD, DC, L.Ac., Ph.D. (Acu.)
Developer of NAET
September 2019

Part 1

Introduction

Hello and welcome to my book *Clarity*. I'm so excited that you've picked up this book to begin your journey of healing from the inside out. Whether you've picked up this book to heal yourself or to hopefully inspire someone else to keep up the good fight, you'll be sure to find something valuable to start a journey of true discovery within these pages.

First, I want to share my story with you so that you can get a better sense of what I went through and why I decided to write this book in the first place. The first part of the book is a deep dive into my personal story. This is necessary to build a framework of what my life was like so you can follow along with the layout in the second part. Then as you continue reading through the chapters, you'll find all the ways that I explored to heal my own condition. I've included several steps I took that you can do as well. My hope is that as you read through the chapters, you'll find information in here that will motivate and inspire you to try some of these methods or, at least, go out in the world and find your own cure. From my experience, since you're already here and reading this book, you've already started your journey to healing. Well done!

As you read through my story and through the steps I've laid out, I encourage you to keep an open mind and allow your thoughts to stretch to what is possible. You'll find in the pages ahead that emotions and life struggles are directly tied to health conditions that I faced, and possibly that you're facing right now. The healing journey is one to celebrate and to understand that through the journey, you'll discover parts of you that you didn't know existed. This is where the real magic happens and you'll be able to transform yourself from struggle to success! Roll up your sleeves and let's dig into journeying down a path of true discovery.

Chapter 1:
The Beginning of My Story

My story is one that builds and twists, just as life does. I didn't realize that my life was so intertwined with my emotions of positive and negative events in my life. I always knew that I was invested in my emotions, since I was easily affected if things didn't go right. However, I had no idea of the extent that my emotions and trauma had on the inner wellbeing. Even though I could get through life with a smile on my face, my insides were a twist of darkness that sat heavily on my heart. I wasn't always this way, but a few years of trauma will do that to anyone. It wasn't until my unfortunate event, where I was forced to look blindness in the eye and say, "not today," that I realized how powerful I really was. I found strength within me and beat a disease that was so rare, my doctors were speechless. But, before we get into all of that, let's start from the beginning of where things went wrong.

I'm just a small-town girl from a place called Minocqua, Wisconsin, or some people like to call it The Northwoods. It's a quiet town where most people travel to in order to get away from the hustle and bustle of the cities. So, really, there isn't too much excitement or busyness that goes on day to day. However, I was beyond busy and stressed out even in this beautiful part of the country. My story starts back in 2013. At the time, my husband and I had owned a martial arts school where I taught women's fitness classes for eight years. We also had just recently bought my parents' house to call our own for our family of four. Our girls were ages one

Clarity

and three, and I just found out that I was pregnant with our third baby. We were so excited to be adding to our family again, but that didn't come without a moment of panic on how I was going to handle three kids and a business that needed my full-time attention. Not to mention, right after I found out I was expecting, I realized I didn't have the right insurance coverage in place to pay for the new baby. At this point in my life, I handled stress decently, but all of the newness of life and adversity of paying for the new baby coming, pushed me into feeling different emotions that started to weigh on me in more ways than I was comfortable with. I started feeling emotions of panic and worry to the point where I felt like I had bricks on my shoulders.

Literally, my new emotions took over and this new transformed Superwoman came out of me from deep within. I started making phone calls to see what insurance coverage I could qualify for now that I was already pregnant. I also kicked my hobby of photography up into a full-blown business in order to put my financial worries in check. My emotions about finances drove me to find a solution. The stress became my driving force to fix this futuristic financial problem.

Nine weeks into my pregnancy, my stress was catapulted higher when I started to spot. When my doctor told me that the baby was fine but my body was doing harm to baby, I realized the stress I was putting on myself was causing the spotting. After some good bedrest and realizing I needed to slow down, everything healed and all was good in my world.

Things were going decently well at this point. I had found delivery coverage for our little bean growing inside of me, and I was finally starting to feel like I could emerge from the stress. Unfortunately, this feeling of bliss didn't last very long. Our 20-week ultrasound appointment was an exciting day, until the doctors saw something on the image that detected a spinal issue with our son. With the lack of proper imagery, the doctor sent me home saying "We can't recreate the image of the vertebrae in question, so you'll have to wait until you deliver for us to do an x-ray on the baby to see what is actually going on. It's possible that it was just a shadow and nothing is wrong as well." Not exactly what a mother wants to hear.

The heavy negative emotions kicked in again full force and Superwoman emerged from deep inside of me again. I started taking wedding jobs with my photography business and trying to figure out any way possible to stash enough cash in case the worst situation happened. I was so worried that we would have a lifetime of medical problems for our son and I couldn't just sit back without feeling prepared. No matter how much my family told me to slow down, I couldn't.

After months of worrying for the outcome with our son's spine, he finally came into the world two weeks early. He was perfect in every way, but, unfortunately, life threw us a curve ball again. After delivering him in our local hospital, he was rushed in an ambulance to a N.I.C.U. hospital three hours from home where they ran tests to see why he couldn't breathe without support. I was devastated and in shock when they took my son, and left me in the hospital to sit and wait to be discharged. My mind was wandering everywhere, like a ping-pong ball bouncing on the sides of my skull, but my body felt paralyzed to move or to talk. This was the first time that I had felt emotions so strong that I couldn't move.

The rollercoaster of emotions overwhelmed me, and the strength of the worry and heartbreak went from paralysis to suddenly Superwoman emerging with a new cape. After gaining my strength, I left the hospital only hours after giving birth. My mother-in-law, Teresa drove me down to the hospital that my son was at to help him heal in any way that I could.

After two weeks of living out of hotels and worrying to the max for his health, we were able to bring our sweet boy home. With lots of support from the N.I.C.U staff, he was given the time he needed for his lungs to grow and strengthen, since he was born so early.

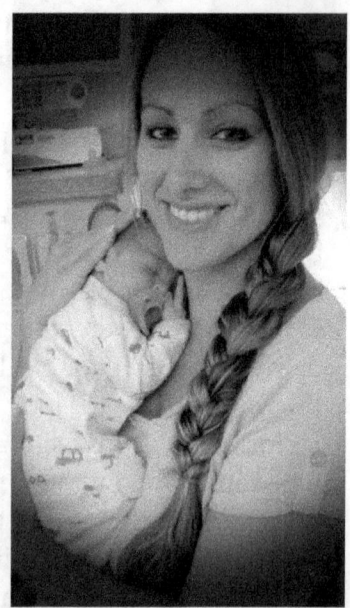

Photo Caption: Nikki Engels holds her son Destin Engels for the first time after two weeks of N.I.C.U. treatment.

Clarity

And to our amazement, his x rays showed that his spine was perfectly fine. Even with this wonderful news, the trauma of the last few weeks left me feeling uncomfortable about his future respiratory health.

While our son was in the N.I.C.U., my husband had also been negotiating deals on buying a new building for our martial arts school. To be honest, this part was such a blur to me, because I was so focused on all of the medical problems with our son, that I just trusted that my husband had the sale handled. Buying the building came at a really bad time, but when you own your own business, time stops for no one. Regardless of the timing, we bought the building and started the remodeling phase.

Two months later, things were going pretty well. I had my son at home and he was thriving. Our family of five was excited to build a new life with our very own martial arts building. While doing the remodeling, we realized all of our dreams were coming true. Things were moving in the right direction and I started to relax a bit, now that all the pieces had perfectly fallen into place over the last few months.

On November 18, 2013, I had gotten the last coverage explanation of the insurance saying our son's medical bills were all taken care of. This was a huge sigh of relief. I felt like the weight of the world had been lifted off of me. Even though I had the okay from the insurance company about the pregnancy, I was still a bit worried about the N.I.C.U. bills. While I was pregnant, I had found an amazing person to help me get the coverage I needed at just the right time. To this day, I'll be forever grateful for this lady, whom I never met in person, for her extra work on my case. Without her help, we would have been buried in medical debt. But, this day was a day that I sighed with relief and was extremely happy to let the financial worry go.

That afternoon, my mother-in-law came over to help me clean up the house. We were folding clothes, I was taking care of paperwork, and the kids were happily playing. It was a wonderful day. We had been so busy remodeling the school the last few weeks that it was nice to catch up on some housework. After we finished, we packed up the kids, and told them we were headed to the library before our oldest had martial arts class with my husband. They were so excited as we packed up our things and left for the evening.

My happy didn't stick around very long. Class had just started for our oldest daughter and the phone rang at the school. It was my mother, who lived right behind our house. She frantically said "Nik, your house is on fire!" I about dropped the phone from shock. I grabbed my husband, who was teaching a class at the time, and we frantically left to see what remained of our beloved home. I remember driving there thinking, *This can't be happening, this can't be happening!* Superwoman took over again and the adrenaline rush made me try to jump out of the truck and run down my driveway. My husband grabbed my wrist as I was about to jump out, but it was all I wanted to do to release some of the emotions that I felt. Shock and panic hit my heart as I realized how angry I was at the universe. "How could this be happening!" I yelled out loud.

As my husband kept me in the truck, we pulled down the long driveway and sure enough, the house was up in flames. The fire department was working so hard to save any part of the house that they could, but when the fireplace fell into the basement, it was a total loss. I was devastated. We were literally homeless in a matter of minutes. As I watched, I stood there yelling and crying. I realized I had left all of the kids' baby books, pictures, and my computer on the dining room table.

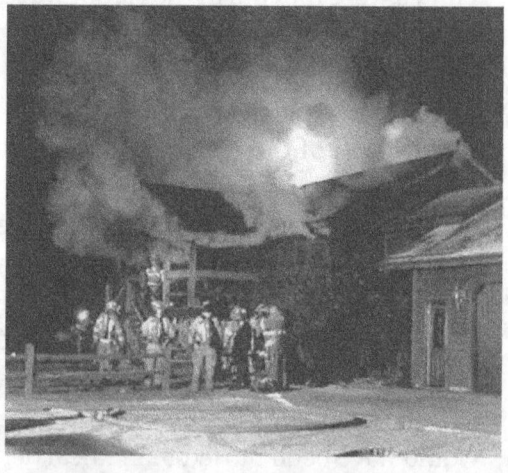

(Photo Caption: Photo captures the Engels home lit up by flames bursting through the roof, while the local fire departments strategize a plan to put it out. Photo taken by Dean Hall, from The Lakeland Times in Minocqua, WI.)

I just fell to my knees, helpless. I was working on updating all of their baby books that morning and didn't put them away. In my head I was angry with myself for not putting them back into our fire safe. My husband held me up as we watched our home burn

Clarity

down to the ground. There was nothing we could do other than stand there and watch. The flames threw orange and yellow bursts of light out of the roof, the smoke billowed out along the fascia, and the fire departments ran around like ants trying to make any progress possible against the beast of a fire.

Fortunately, we had homeowner's insurance and were put up in a hotel until we could find a place to rent. That first night was extremely painful and sad, trying to explain to the girls, who were now four and two, what had happened. They didn't understand why we couldn't go home and they cried for their beloved possessions. Ironically, our older daughter left her favorite baby doll at home that day. Trying to explain to her that she couldn't see her again, felt like we were explaining death to her for the first time. It was beyond painful to see her hurting just as we were. But again, my husband and I tried to remind the kids that we were all okay. We were safe, and our dog was safe, thanks to my father who had gotten her out. We had to remind ourselves that we could put the pieces back together again and rebuild a house. I found comfort in that, but my emotions and stress levels were through the roof. My body felt every emotion as if I were being physically attacked, and my mind was spinning like a top.

Life looked extremely crazy at this point. We literally were getting shuffled from rental house to rental house due to weird leasing agreements at that time of the year, while remodeling an old building and trying to turn it into a gem for our martial arts school, and having a newborn who kept getting sick and was now struggling to keep his airways open. In the midst of having our world turned upside down, we had to sanely decide what our new house would look like while working with the insurance adjusters on the payments. I was, for lack of better words, a hot mess! I was such a hot mess that all I kept saying was, "I can't breathe… I feel like something is going to blow inside of me." Night after night, I would sit in my truck before pulling into our rental house's tiny garage, crying. The tears poured out of my eyes, as I felt like my world was coming down on me. My anxiety, fear, and powerlessness were pushing me to a place that I didn't like and that wasn't comfortable. Where did that happy girl go who was inside of me? Was she gone forever? I was afraid to know the answer as I sat and cried. I feared that she would never return. The amount of emotions I had felt with our son's health and the house fire made me feel like I was drowning in a sea of negativity.

Slowly, our life was being put back together physically. But that didn't help the stress between my husband and me. We were both dealing with the stress differently, and were having a hard time putting down our imaginary swords. We were there for each other, but there was distance and arguments as there would be with any couple who had gone through so much. We did the best we could to find time for each other though, and we celebrated our wins along the way as much as we could. However, our hearts were hurting in different ways, and we both needed time to heal.

I knew my husband needed to get away to clear his head and heal in his own way. I called a mutual martial arts friend who lived in Portland, Oregon and asked if my husband could come out by him for a week. I was hoping if Gary visited his martial arts school that he would find a happy spark of inspiration and positivity that he could bring home to our family and to the students at our school. After a lot of coaxing, Gary finally agreed to go. On my way home from dropping him off at the airport, I got another frustrating call. One of our black belt students had stopped at the martial arts academy to grab something. To her amazement the school was filled with water. I again was in shock as I heard her hesitantly tell me what was happening as she stood in the school. *How am I going to deal with this mess?* I thought as I literally just dropped my husband off at the airport.

I drove the hour home in complete turmoil. I had no idea what I would be walking into or how I would fix it all. I was certain of one thing; I had only six days to get it cleaned up so that when my husband came back, we could continue on with business as usual. Somehow, I magically had to figure it out while caring for a newborn, a two-year-old, and a four-year-old. My head was spinning. My emotional and physical pain was encompassing my entire body again.

I slowly drove into the parking lot and saw, to my amazement, about 30 people helping to clean up the mess. Most of

Clarity

them were on the roof shuffling off snow. As I walked into the building, I heard multiple voices and vacuums. The melting roof water had literally been going down the roof drain and had backed up through the water fountain. It was just spewing out at a constant stream of forceful water. I stood there for a minute not knowing what to do. The water was so thick that it was dripping through the floor and into the basement from the electrical outlets. I felt like time stood still as I watched everyone around me work. I ended up breaking down and just stood there and cried as our black belt student came up to me and gave me a hug. How in the world was I going to fix this!? My world was crashing down once again.

Finally, things slowed down and everyone went home. I called the insurance company and luckily things all worked out to have the floors and carpets cleaned. Unfortunately, our coverage wouldn't cover all the other water damage that had happened. I did the best I could with what I had. I rolled up all the martial arts flooring, cleaned it, and stood it up to dry with huge industrial fans blowing on it. The rest had to wait until my husband came home. It was another devastating blow, but, somehow, I was able to pull it all together in order to have classes when my husband came back.

About a year later, the house was finished and we had fixed our newly remodeled school from the flood. Things were looking up. We took two years to settle into our new environments, but one thing that didn't change was our sore hearts and our son's breathing health. He was sick all the time and needed constant care for his lungs. For some reason, every time he would get sick, his breathing was a fight to control. Most of my time was spent on keeping him healthy. My stress from worrying about him was out of control and caused me to not fully take care of myself in the way that I needed. My Superwoman self would come out and take care of business to make sure everyone else was happy and healthy. My husband and sisters were worried about me, as they could see that I was wearing myself thin. But, I would reassure them that I was alright and the worst was behind me. It felt like I was lying to them. But what choice did I have? I had to be strong for them and take care of things. There weren't any excuses. I always tried to have the attitude of, "Let me roll my sleeves up, and I'll dig into the mess and sort it out."

My husband and I continued on trying to create more businesses and opportunities for our family. We wanted to leave all the pain in our past and build an even better future. We ended up buying an old coffee hut and turned it into a fully functional drive-up coffee shop; we took on training other students who wanted to take their martial arts to a competitive level in the fighting ring; we expanded our martial arts program to another town; and I continued taking photography jobs. People would come up to me and ask, "How are you doing all of this?" And my answer was always, "I don't know!"

Inside, I was crumbling; I was physically and emotionally beat up. I hadn't really healed from the traumas I had experienced over the last few years. My husband and I both thought that if we pushed harder and worked harder, that all the pain would go away. But, it honestly didn't. That pain festered and grew inside me like a cancer. Things around me were going faster than I could keep up with, and it was creating that feeling of "something's going to blow" even more. I was drowning in my own misery.

I knew something had to change, but it was beyond my control at this point. The businesses, the people, the long daily to-do lists were all in full swing, and I couldn't stop any of it. My world was rotating around me and I was in denial, thinking that I could keep running this race against what my body was screaming. My body and mind wanted to slow down, but I saw no way to get off the rapidly spinning hamster wheel.

Meanwhile, as my world was rapidly spinning around me, I decided to get ready for a Jiu Jitsu tournament. It was my first Jiu Jitsu tournament! I was scared out of my mind, yet I had this drive inside of me to push hard in class. I trained with some of the biggest and toughest men in class. They were getting ready for their competitive level fights in the ring, and I was their conditioning coach. I was and still am a smaller lady, weighing no more than 115 pounds, so I had to train even harder to keep up. That added a whole additional layer of stress to my already long lists of roles in my life. In class, I pushed through sweat, blood, and sometimes tears. I didn't want to show weakness, especially against these pro fighters. For goodness sake, I was one of their coaches, so I often ignored my

Clarity

body screaming at me to stop. I was mentally focused on getting ready for this competition because I didn't want to get my butt handed to me. Physically however, I was hurting and I felt the walls of physical fatigue closing in on me.

During one of the last practices before the tournament, I was rolling with one of the fighters. When I went to escape a position, I felt a sudden stabbing pain in my right side and lower back area. I didn't know what hit me, but it felt like my insides were being shredded apart. I immediately stopped and my rolling partner asked what was wrong. I couldn't even explain what had happened, and I was so confused because I was never in a dangerous position. All I knew was that my body was sending out signals to alert me to slow down and heal. Unfortunately, I didn't listen. I mean, I had a tournament to get ready for. I wasn't going to make a fool of myself at my very first tournament. I was going to win. I had something to prove to myself, and I had to prove to everyone else that I was mentally and physically tough. After that night of practice, I still couldn't put my finger on what was wrong with my right side. It wasn't really my spine, but the pain was radiating outward from my right side somewhere. It hurt to walk and it hurt to twist. Yet, I pushed through it anyways and continued to teach and train.

The tournament day came and went with a very disappointing loss. My back never fully recovered, and competing in the tournament made it worse. I stuck it out as long as I could, but I ended up in the worst position possible for my back and had to tap out of the match. I was devastated afterwards, even though my teammates told me that I did a really good job for my first match. I felt like I had lost control of my body. I was hurting physically, mentally, and emotionally. I felt numb to all things other than the pain. I really couldn't figure out what was wrong with my back or how it happened in the first place. Nothing added up in my mind, and the spinning thoughts of trying to figure out this puzzle only frustrated me more. The anger grew inside of me like bubbling lava about to burst everywhere. I was mad at the situation, at my body, and the universe. It was as if that loss was more than just the match. It signified all the heartache and struggles that accumulated over the years. I had lost me. I lost who I used to be.

After a few weeks went by, I started to notice other things happening to my body alongside the constant physical pain and extreme exhaustion. I started to develop what I now know were food sensitivities. I would eat a meal, any meal, and my stomach would blow up to looking like I was three months pregnant. After training with the fighters for almost a year, I was approaching a six pack, which I was pretty darn proud of after having three kids. Suddenly, all of that changed. My body was shifting before my eyes and I again felt like I was losing control. I couldn't pinpoint why my body was reacting to food all of a sudden. I started to think about my physical structure, and the thought had crossed my mind that it could be possible that my spine was out of line. Maybe I needed to have it adjusted? I wasn't all that excited about seeing a chiropractor, but, if it helped the pain and now my potbelly, then by all means I was up for anything. I didn't have the time or patience to figure this problem out on my own, so I took a leap and contacted a chiropractor who I knew quite well to help.

I was so optimistic that morning of my chiropractic appointment. Finally, I was going to get the answers that I needed, and I would be pain free and ready to run ahead of my spinning, crazy, circus of a life again. As much as I wanted to get off the hamster wheel, the fast-paced life weirdly thrilled the superhero inside of me. I figured a few appointments and I would be good to go on taking charge and living large again. As fate would have it, that wasn't the plan for me.

I left my appointment with a fuzzy idea of what was wrong. It seemed like my x-rays showed my back wasn't as aligned as I had hoped. The chiropractor's pessimistic view of my back made me feel hopeless. He suggested that I should wear inserts in my shoes even during my workouts, and that I would need adjustments quite frequently to fix the pain. I wasn't exactly thrilled to hear the news, but I was hopeful that his plan would work. After a few appointments of being adjusted throughout my lower spine, I really wasn't getting any better. The pain was still there and I was getting frustrated that this process was taking as long as it was.

Around the beginning of March 2015, I went in for another adjustment. The chiropractor suggested that I needed to have my neck adjusted. I was hesitant, only because the idea of it scared me. But, I was dedicated to feeling better. I tried to lie calmly on the table as he had my head in his hands. I kept telling myself, *It will be fine, it will be fine,* and before I knew it, it was over. He had cracked my neck and I was good to go. Yet, I left the office not quite feeling like myself. I got home and I was physically hurting everywhere. I ran to the bathroom and took my temperature and sure enough I had a fever. My family was sick earlier in the week, but I wasn't ill before I left for my appointment that morning. The fever came out of nowhere and hit me violently.

Trying to deal with the fever was one thing, but I couldn't control how much pain I was in all throughout my body. I couldn't sleep, I couldn't move, and I couldn't stop crying from the pain I was suddenly in. I had plenty of fevers in my days, and I knew what those aches and pains felt like. This was like someone was cutting nerves in my whole body, and then letting me lie there and suffer with them all exposed. I lay on the couch crying from nerve pain shooting down into my feet. At one point, I grabbed my son's golf balls from his room. Shoving them into points on my hips while I lay on top of them seemed to ease some of the pain traveling downward. I was crawling out of my skin, yet there was no letting up; the pain was constant and agonizing.

The intense pain went on for days. Things started to finally let up slightly after about a week, at least to the point where I could function in my daily tasks. I tried teaching my women's fitness class, but I was struggling to feel my feet. The nerve pain was taking over and my feet were in and out of sensation, so much so, that I often tripped in class because I couldn't feel the ground. I was scared, and again confused as to what was happening with my body. I was angry again and I couldn't stop crying from the constant ache of nerve pain. A few weeks after my life changing adjustment, the nerve pain wasn't only traveling down my legs, but had also extended into my arms and fingers and throughout my lower abdomen. My belly felt like I had hot coals directly on my skin, just burning their way through me. I was physically cold, but my whole body always felt like it was lit on fire from constant nerve pain inside. Emotionally, I was lost. Questions repeatedly ran through my head. I was angry with myself for going down this road with the chiropractor to begin with. If I had only listened to that small voice inside that said, *Don't do a neck adjustment,* then maybe I wouldn't be in this awful position now. *Ahhh!* was all I could say in my head!

I finally got to the point where I knew I needed help and going back to the chiropractor at this point wasn't the answer. I called a local physical therapist and explained to them what had happened. They schedule my appointment immediately. I was surprised by their rush to get me in. I was expecting to have to wait a few months before they would be able to see me. This worried me a bit that they got me into their schedule days after I had called. But, I felt some relief in knowing that maybe I would finally get some answers on how to dig myself out of this hole.

My first appointment wasn't what I expected. I was immediately rushed to have an MRI taken of my spine. The physical therapist was concerned that I had multiple sclerosis and he couldn't help me until he really knew what was going on inside of me. I about lost my emotional poise when they suggested that it could be even more severe than I thought. Reluctantly, I went alone to my MRI appointment. I felt alone and scared, but I also didn't want to be around anyone. My emotional pain was so thick that I didn't want to drag anyone down with me. A million thoughts ran through my head as I lay in the MRI tube on a cold, sterile table to wait for my fate.

Fortunately, the results came back and I was totally okay! I didn't have any signs of MS and my spine looked good. Finally, good news! I felt like I had dodged a very fast speeding bullet. I instantly felt like I could breath, but that still didn't answer why I had nerve pain and why I was still hurting everywhere. My physical therapist put me on a schedule to come in a few times a week to work on my body's issues. At the same time, I was scratching for answers.

I reluctantly dragged myself back to the chiropractor to have a sit-down meeting with him. I explained what had happened since I left my last appointment with him, as best as I could, and then proceeded to ask him what went wrong. He was shocked, and I was taken aback by his emotions that he was trying so hard to hold in. He sheepishly told me that he didn't know what happened. He explained that he did everything he was supposed to according to his training. At that moment, I was so angry and hurt by him. I knew this man, and I trusted him. I didn't understand the whole situation and why I couldn't find the answers that I so desperately needed in that moment.

In hindsight, this chiropractor didn't do anything wrong. He had no way of seeing what my body was going through at that time. My body was crumbling from within and neither of us knew the extent of it. At the time, I felt like it was his fault that my body was now worse than when I started. After learning so much over the last few years, I truly believe he didn't do anything wrong. He did what he knew, but he didn't realize how fragile my system was in that moment. Also, my immune system was fighting off an illness my family had just had. While I still don't agree or feel comfortable with neck adjustments, I'd like to state that I don't put fault on him in any way.

Three months have gone by at this time and I have been diligently going to my physical therapy appointments. I looked forward to the little relief that they gave each time I went, but overall, I still had nerve pain, chronic fatigue, food allergies, and my back/side area still throbbed with pain. The appointments at least helped me continue with my normal daily activities, but I still didn't feel like myself. I was starting to learn how to live with daily pain as a normal aspect of life.

On Monday, July 4, 2016, business was running as usual. Little did I know, I was approaching on the biggest shifting point in my life. Yes, it was a holiday. However, it also meant we had to work extra hard at our businesses. The coffee shop was buzzing and needed to be managed. It was a struggling business to keep the cash flow coming in. Since we lived in a tourist town, the holiday was the best way to recoup some of the costs from staying open during the slow winter. We were also getting ready to participate in the 4th of July town parade. Our martial arts school participated to celebrate and to hopefully inspire new students to join our academy. Our family was like little busy bees running around making everything happen. It was crunch time, making every minute count. We checked our list: a) Was the coffee shop stocked? b) How were the employees? c) Is the float ready to go? d) Does everyone have their uniforms for the parade? etc., etc. The list went on and on.

Now, I also have to give you a little background at this time. Starting from April 2016 to July 2016, not only was business in full swing while my health was declining, but I was also having a difficult time with my extended family. There wasn't much dialogue between my parents and me other than frustration and anger. From what I've experienced, most families have some difficult times just like this, but my situation was an ongoing battle over the years. We had good times and we had bad times. July 4th, 2016 was at the height of a really bad battle of which I didn't see an end.

My husband pulled into the parking lot of the baseball field, waiting to get in line with all of the other businesses for the parade. I was excited! It was a lot of work to be in the parade, but it was also a lot of fun. We had a great group of kids and adults joining us this year, and we had a great demo figured out too. It was a beautiful sunny day and the spirit and enthusiasm was all around us. All of that excitement and free-spirited behavior I had went right out the window when my husband said, "Nik, your parents are right in front of us." I went into a panic. I looked at them and then back at my husband. "What?!" They're never here. I looked and realized they were helping out with another business's float. I was shocked. I jumped out of the truck after it was parked and didn't know what to do. I was so afraid that my parents and I would have an argument right in front of all of our students and the townspeople. I didn't really know what to think or how to act. I needed to stay focused on what I had to do in that moment, but my emotions were hanging out of my body like clothing flapping in the wind on a clothesline.

I started to decorate the truck as best as I could, but my hands were shaking and my head couldn't clearly think. I was trying to tie on martial art belts in a specific way around the doors and windows of the truck and I honestly couldn't do it. A friend came over and asked if I needed help. He could see that I was struggling, but he didn't know what was going on. I tried and tried to tie the belt on right and then I realized my hands were shaking too hard to make the knot. My friend took over and I tried to gather myself.

Clarity

"What was wrong with me?" I kept repeating to myself, "Just get it together!" Yet my body was doing its own thing and I couldn't get a grip. Seeing my parents had literally pushed me over an edge that I didn't even see coming. The disturbing thing was, they didn't even do anything wrong in that moment. They never said a word or came over to our section; they didn't do anything, yet my body literally felt like it was being attacked. I couldn't breathe, my body felt tingly, and I felt revved up. I could have run a marathon at that moment from all of the adrenaline that was dumped into my system. Somehow, I had to gather myself and shove the fear I had somewhere else before the parade and fast!

We decided that on our float, I would demonstrate a Jiu Jitsu self-defense sequence. I partnered with another student who knew the moves well. Things were going great during the parade. Somehow just moving and demonstrating the techniques helped my body relax a bit. At first, I was a little fuzzy with the techniques, but, soon, I started to feel my body normalize again. As we demonstrated, one of my training partner's legs had hit me in the side of the head. I felt a little dizzy afterwards, but it wasn't anything to be alarmed about. I had hit my head harder getting out of my truck on occasion, so it wasn't anything that worried me.

In fact, I felt so much better after the parade from just the movements of the demo that my slight headache didn't bother me at all. The headache was better than the shaky, revved up feeling I had earlier. Moving had pushed out the adrenaline and helped put my body back to a more

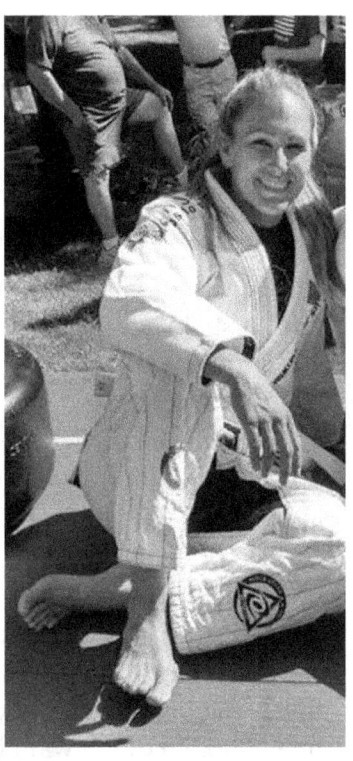

(Photo Caption: Nikki taking a quick photo before her Jiu Jitsu demonstration on July 4, 2016. This picture was the last photo taken before the retinal bleed attacked her eye.)

normalized state. Yet, my mind was still laser focused on the family issues at hand. In my head, I was struggling with thoughts of confusion, anger, hurt, and feeling misunderstood by my family. I didn't know what to do with all of the emotions and it led me to stay on a constant hamster wheel of negativity once again.

The next day, I was back to classes and our regular work schedule, yet my mind was still fixated on seeing my family the day before. The emotions of fear, anxiety, anger, and more had rocked me to a level that I couldn't have understood at that time. I tried to relax my mind that morning by doing some gardening. Later, I went into our academy to teach my fitness program. After class, I had a conversation with my youngest sister Karlie and told her that I was struggling with my contacts.

All day long, I felt like I was looking through saran wrap. She asked if my contacts were new and I told her I had put new ones in right before I left to teach class. I thought I had gotten dirt in them from gardening in the morning. But, I still felt like something was wrong with my vision in my right eye. I asked her, "Do you think someone could just lose their vision overnight?" And she responded "No! Not at your age." So I took comfort in that, since I was only 32 at the time, and I went home. *She was probably right,* I thought. *I must just be stressed from the parade the day before and I needed to get some good sleep.*

Wednesday, July 6th my vision was getting worse. I kept looking in my eye to see if there was something in it. Maybe a hair, a piece of dirt, anything! But nothing was there. I even asked my husband repeatedly to check my eye. And every time he said, "I don't see anything." In my gut, I knew something was wrong, seriously wrong. I stayed up for a few hours after everyone went to bed to finish editing some photos I had just taken from a recent photoshoot. I didn't want to be irresponsible and not have these jobs done if life handed me another challenge the next day. When I finally lay down in bed at 2:00 a.m., I realized I was having trouble sleeping because I kept seeing a white light when I closed my eyes. I knew in my heart this wasn't good!

I sent a text message to my other sister, Malina, who happened to work at an eye clinic. I told her what I was experiencing

Clarity

and to just call me when she got to work. I struggled to go to bed, but I was hoping I would just need some eye drops and all would be totally fine. I woke up to my phone ringing at 6:30 am. I was so frustrated with my sister as I messaged her back, instead of answering my phone. I snapped, telling her I had been up all night working and I just wanted to sleep. I asked her to just schedule me in later in the afternoon. Her response was, "Nope, get out of bed and go shower. I already put you in the schedule at 8:00 am with Dr. Ben Redman." She was calm and bossy all at the same time. Ohhh, how the rage in me swelled! I was irritated that I had to do this in the first place and boiling mad that I had to get up so early. Little did I know, she knew what was going on and was pushing me to get there as fast as possible.

I arrived at the clinic, grumpy and pissed off on July 7, 2016. I was tired, emotional, and, to be honest, scared. Thoughts of *Now what mess am I going to have to deal with?* popped in my head. At this point in life, I expected the other shoe to drop and for life to give me another problem that Superwoman was going to have to fix. However, even though I was engulfed with emotions, it couldn't have prepared me for the life lesson I was about to get.

I sat in the cold air-conditioned room after having what seemed like a million pictures taken of the inside of my eye. No one was saying anything about my condition yet. As I sat there trying to make out things around me with my fuzzy vision, I felt my gut screaming that trouble was on the way. I tried to push it down, but the feeling just overwhelmed me.

Dr. Redman walked in. We had gone to high school together years ago, so it was nice to see a familiar face. He looked extremely professional with his dark hair styled slightly to the side and his white coat hugging him. Unfortunately, as great as it was to reunite, I could see on his meek, expressionless face that his news for me wasn't good. He tried to use an upbeat and positive voice as he showed me the images that had just been taken of my right eye. He said, "Nikki, It looks like you have a bleed in your retina. The fluid is pooling in your eye and is starting to expand to the center of your vision. If it pushes to the middle of your eye, you could lose your sight in that eye forever." As the words came out of his mouth, the cold chair around me felt like it was squeezing me from all sides. I couldn't breathe out of fear and anxiety.

I finally croaked out a sound and asked, "So I just need some drops or something, right?" He looked concerned and again tried to use a happy tone to soften the blow. "We're going to have to send you to a specialist who will do an injection in your eye to stop the bleeding. The medication will allow for the fluid to go down and save your sight." Fear and anger rose up inside me as I asked, "What?! A needle in my eye? Like literally they're going to put a needle in my eye?" I started to ramble, "So this has to be from getting hit in the head at the parade, right?! How does this happen to someone? This is unreal!" His sweet eyes looked at me as he said, "It's possible, but we aren't sure. The ophthalmologist, Dr. Stewart (not his real name), will know more about what's going on with your condition. For now, we need to schedule you and try to get you in with him as soon as possible, so that this doesn't cause permanent damage." I think at this point he was reassuring me that everything would be okay, but I had a moment of Charlie Brown's teacher and all I heard was the low muffles of his voice.

He left the room to make the call and I sat there dazed. I was all alone in the room. On one hand, I preferred that so I could process what was just told to me. On the other hand, I wanted my husband to hold me and tell me I was going to be alright. The cold, air-conditioned room didn't feel frigid anymore. I was sweating with anger, confusion, and fear

I didn't have the best history with needles due to being hospitalized for asthma as a child, so the idea of a needle in my eye was tremendously terrifying. I looked over at the image on the computer screen. It looked like a huge bubbling blob of black liquid threatening to invade my vision like an oil spill in the ocean. Just slowly creeping and spreading in any direction that it wanted to go.

Clarity

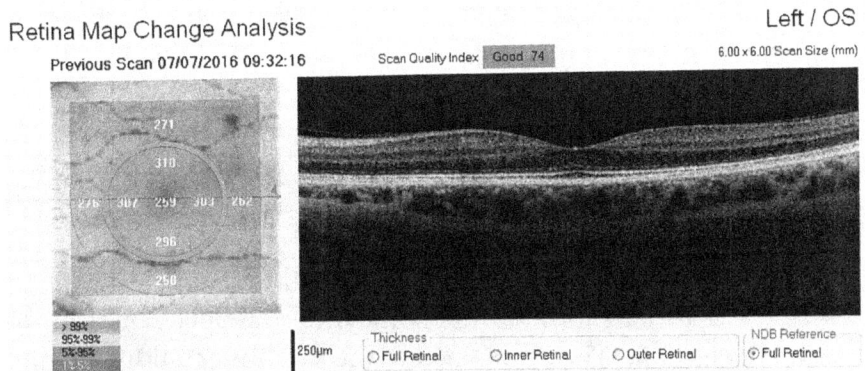

(Photo Caption: This is an OTC Scan of the left "good" eye. The nice white curves are how the retina should appear. The numbers to the left are in the normal range.)

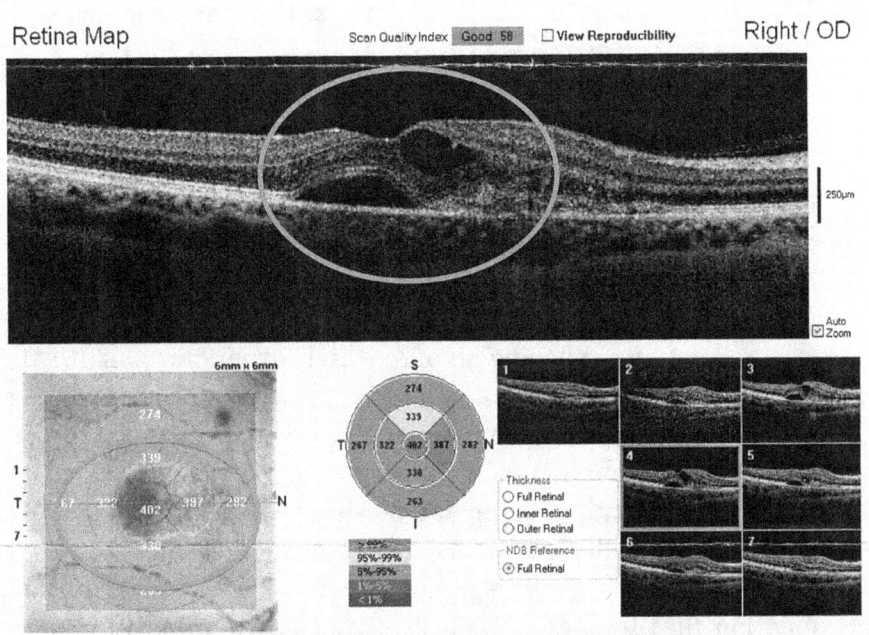

(Photo Caption: This is an OTC scan of the right eye with the retinal bleed. The black holes in the white lines are blood and fluid pooling in the back of the eye. The fluid is encroaching in on the center of my vision. The numbers to the left, show the thickness of the retina.)

Immediately I thought in a sarcastic tone, *How are you going to get out of this one Superwoman?* Superwoman was really starting to get on my nerves. I hated the idea that she would creep up in my head. I wanted her to go away. I wanted to have a nice, quiet, and peaceful life. Why did I feel that it was up to me, aka Superwoman, to fix every traumatizing situation? And now this time, it was me, actually me who was falling apart. How does that strong inner voice, that Superwoman, fix this mess! How?!

My thoughts were interrupted by the doctor and his staff coming back in. They explained to me that they couldn't get me in see the retinal specialist until Tuesday. It was only Thursday! I had to wait all weekend, and into the next week! The staff started to explain to me the restrictions that I was on. In a sympathetic voice, the sweet tech said, "You'll have to be on bed rest over the weekend. You can't do any heavy lifting and try not to bend over where your head is down. Take it easy and try and relax until you can get in with Dr. Stewart." I was in shock! I could hear the words she was saying, but my mind was somewhere else.

I felt like my body was just going through the motions, but my mind was whizzing from the past day's events to futuristic visions of what I was going to have to do. I also started thinking about my long to-do list. Work wasn't going to wait and my list was never ending. It seems so silly now to be putting work ahead of my health, but at that moment, work was less painful than the news I had just gotten.

As if I were having an out-of-body experience, I slowly took the loose papers of information from the tech and made my way out into the waiting room where my sister worked in optical. She looked at me, and I numbingly looked back at her. She saw the papers in my hand and, with a loving and concerned expression, said, "Let's go outside and talk." As we made our way to the front door, my legs were weak, my hands were tingling, and my body was lit with a fiery emotion that I couldn't control. Anger at life flowed through my veins as I could feel Superwoman taking over again. My sister calmly said, "It'll be okay. Lots of people have to get shots like that for macular degeneration."

Clarity

Her words and her expression didn't match, and I boastfully came back with harshness and evasion. "I can't believe I have to wait until Tuesday. Dez [my son] has an allergy appointment an hour and a half away on Monday. I can't miss that! Since I couldn't get in with Dr. Stewart tomorrow, I had to push my appointment until Tuesday. Dez's breathing isn't great and his appointment has to come first. This can wait until afterwards." I thought my sister was going to punch me in the face. She answered back with, "You do know this is serious, right?! You'll be fine to wait until Tuesday for your appointment and go to Dez's appointment on Monday, but you do need to take it easy this weekend to keep it from getting worse. Everything else can wait!" I was furious! But, she was right. It was only one shot; I should be okay. The moment of bravery hovered for a few minutes. Having my sister answer my anger back with compassion and fierceness amazingly calmed me to realize she was right. I got in my truck after a long hug from her and drove home, using my good eye to lead the way. Even though it's legally acceptable and I was safe to drive with one eye, it was still out of my comfort zone.

That weekend was a total blur of emotions. My husband had organized a group of friends to help pour concrete on our raised deck that we had built over the summer. It was the last piece to finish the project and I was nervous about the cost and how it was really going to come together. Since my latest news from the eye doctors, I was ordered to stay inside and not to help with any of the outside concrete work. Malina came over to the house to help me make food for the crew and she repeatedly was telling me to relax and sit down. Superwoman wouldn't have it! My fury grew from the anxiety of the guys working outside and it amplified my nervousness. At one point, I heard my husband yelling and swearing as the concrete was drying faster than he expected. I was trapped inside, only to pace around, hoping that things would all turn out with the project. We were spending a lot of money to rebuild this part of our home, and I felt guilty that this eye condition condemned me from helping.

By the end of the night of the stressful day, my eye was so painful that it made me nauseous. My eye socket felt as though it was going to explode the black blob of threatening liquid all over the place. My eye was pushing outward and the intense headache came to follow. I had to wear sunglasses in the house to help with the straining bright lights, as our concrete crew stayed over to watch the UFC Fights on TV. At this point, everyone thought my eye was no big deal.

We all figured it was a sports injury and I needed one shot of medicine for it to become a good, quick wound story. My sweet sister, Malina stayed with me the whole time and tried to help relieve the agonizing pain that I was in. She took me in the other room with ice packs and blankets to get away from all the noise and eye distractions. I expressed to her my concerns and worries as my eye was becoming increasingly worse. She helped me become stronger and get my thoughts under control. That moment was so powerful to me because I knew I had her support to navigate through this journey. I found comfort in her words because I was grabbing onto any life saving devices I could.

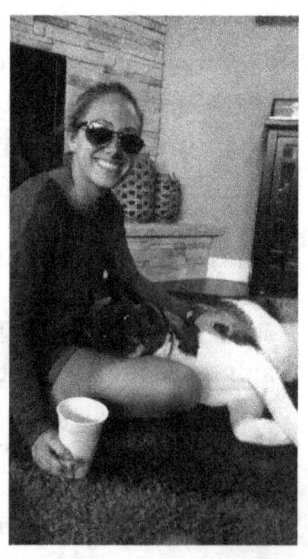

(Photo Caption: Nikki sitting in her living room, wearing sunglasses to help with her vision, while her dog Lanikai consoled her.)

The day finally came for me to see Dr Stewart. Our hour drive felt like a torture ride to make a visit with death. My husband kept trying to be my strong, supportive, rock by telling me that everything was going to be okay. But, in my heart, I was absolutely terrified. Since our appointment was so far away and our kids were so little at the time, we all decided to make the trip together. I wanted them all there to hopefully shed some strength and positivity on me.

We arrived at the large, powerful clinic where the words "Eye" in their logo jumped off the sign as if it itself were the threat. We parked and I entered the building nervously. My eye was throbbing, my heart was pounding from heartache, and my body felt like it was floating along, just going through the motions again. I had to be brave and just face the music with this situation, but every part of me wanted to run out of the door and hide. I looked around and

Clarity

took in the whole view of the clinic. This two-story building felt enormous with walls of glass windows, tall ceilings, and a very sterile color of gray/blue accenting the waiting room walls. The place was buzzing with patients and staff systematically running around each other while they worked on their tasks.

My eye doctors back home had warned me that the crowds of people at this clinic were going to be quite older than I was. From the sounds of it, most of the elderly population had to have eye injections quite frequently due to macular degeneration. Their condition was different than what I had because of my age, but the treatment was relatively the same. I knew this walking in, however, it really hit me when I realized I was amongst a group of people who also had to deal with the same outcome as I did. I stood there, taking it all in, and time stopped. This wasn't right. This wasn't where I thought I'd be at the age of 32.

We were shuffled from waiting room to waiting room as the nurses filtered me in and out for preliminary testing. After some time, I was finally invited to stay in the final waiting room to allow my eyes to dilate from the drops the nurses had just given me. Across from me, an elderly woman accidentally peed on the waiting room chair because she couldn't get up in time to make it to the bathroom. I sat there, holding my kids close, thinking about what I had just witnessed. While my thoughts of sympathy went to that woman, I was struck with a million questions about my situation. Why was I here and why was this happening to me?

This whole situation felt wrong. It was as if I were in a bad dream. I looked around and realized all the elderly patients couldn't keep their eyes off me and my family. I felt exposed, questioned, and utterly embarrassed that I had to be there. I realized they too probably had a bunch of questions as to why such a young family shared this waiting room with them. As I looked around again, I realized that no matter what age everyone was, this fate was hard to deal with. Everyone looked stressed, worried, and distraught, just as I did at that moment.

My thoughts were interrupted when the nurse called me back. We followed her down a hallway that seemed to never end. Each side was lined with different waiting rooms, all filled with patients waiting to see the doctor. I felt like I was a cow being pushed to the slaughter house. My insides twisted and turned with anticipation for what I was going to learn. As she had me look at an Amsler grid, or simple grid paper, I realized the lines were not straight, everything was wavy and it made me nauseous.

Dr. Stewart finally came in after answering multiple questions from his staff. He was a young, hip doctor whose attire matched his smooth personality. He wasn't much older than me, probably mid 30s. His hair was dark, his face charmingly filled with studious glasses, and he had the expression of a concerned friend. I liked the energy he brought in the room. It was bold, confident, yet concerned and sympathetic to my situation. We talked for some time about what I was seeing and feeling and after he did an examination of my eye, he gave me the news I wasn't ready to hear. "Nikki, you have advanced myopic degeneration and neovascular membranes. It's not from a sports-related injury; rather, it's from a rare genetic eye disease. You're at high risk for vision loss because the blood vessel is leaking so closely to the center of your vision."

I looked at my husband and looked back at Dr. Stewart, asking, "Genetic? No one in my family has anything like this. Are you sure it's not a sports-related injury?" I frantically asked the question in hopes that he was wrong. If this weren't a sports injury and if it truly were a disease, did that mean this would be an ongoing condition I'd have to worry about? In my mind, a sports injury meant I needed a one-time shot and I'd be fixed. I was holding onto the comfort of my idea of sports injury to make me feel tough and brave. The words *genetic disease* confronted me with the possibility that this was a doomsday fate, and my eye was aging 40 years faster than it should!

Dr. Stewart responded that my condition looked completely different than a head injury would, and he tried to reassure me that sometimes this just happens in life. He went on to state that this condition wasn't very common, which meant there was a lack of research and data regarding why it happened in the first place. He proceeded to tell me that he had had a small handful of patients around my age, no more than ten, who had gone through the same thing. Some had to have injections for the rest of their lives and some got better after a few treatments. There, unfortunately, weren't any connections between their stories that would suggest any clues to why this was happening to me.

    I was devastated, to say the least. I sat there for a moment asking him if stress could cause this or if somehow my other health problems prior could have been the culprit. His answer was that stress could play a part, but for the most part, they didn't have any research to say that it could or couldn't be the actual cause. This information didn't sit well with me. I wanted answers, something, anything to hang onto that would give some rays of hope for me. I was left feeling like I was grabbing air. I felt like I was trying to grab an imaginary float to save myself from drowning in my own misery.

    I was snapped back into reality when Dr. Stewart started to talk about our treatment plan. I became laser focused on his every word. *Finally, we're getting to the plan,* I thought. And then my heart hit my throat when he started to talk about the injection again. He started to explain that the abnormal growing blood vessel in the back of my eye was causing macular swelling and the buildup of fluid was contributing to the loss of vision. He continued explaining that only a few years prior they didn't have the medication they do now to help with these conditions. Prior to using the injections, they used a technique called Focal Laser Therapy. According to the American Academy of Ophthalmology, "Laser treatment is sometimes used to seal off leaking blood vessels in the retina that are causing macular edema."[1] However, this treatment can cause damage to the central vision as time goes on and more laser treatments are needed. He continued by explaining that the injections were a better way to go so that I wasn't left with permanent black holes in my vision from the laser therapy.

    I was feeling better at this point about the options that I sort of had. One, if I left the condition as it was, I would go blind for sure. Two, if I did the laser treatment I would probably be left with blind spots. Three, I could take an injection in the eye and save my sight. Naturally, the third option was the best choice. He made me feel really good about the injection, but he did also explain that there were some risks. I agreed to move forward, since he seemed so confident and he explained that he did these injections multiple times a day, every day. I found comfort in that, but my hands were cold and clammy as I sat waiting for the event to unfold. I also agreed to let extra staff come into the room to learn how to do the procedure, which, looking back, was a horrible idea.

It felt like as soon as I agreed to the injection, the somber staff suddenly came to life. They were in and out of the room, pulling out equipment, and organizing paperwork that I had to read through and sign. I suddenly became extremely overwhelmed. One of the sheets they had to read to me, since my vision was so poor due to all the dilation drops, as well as my condition, was the "Informed Consent for Avastin™ (Bevacizumab) Intravitreal Injection."[2]

As I was listening to the nurse read through all of the information, I was agreeing that everything I heard from her aligned with what my doctor just stated. Then she read, "Avastin™ was not initially developed to treat your eye condition. Based upon the results of clinical trials that demonstrated its safety and effectiveness, Avastin™ was approved by the Food and Drug Administration (FDA) for the treatment of metastatic colorectal cancer." My mind shot right to pure alarm! "What!? Cancer medication?! Seriously!?" I couldn't believe what I was hearing. I delayed asking my questions until she finished reading the rest of the consent form.

She continued to the next section that explained what the medication did. "Avastin™ works by blocking a substance known as vascular endothelial growth factor or VEGF. Blocking or inhibiting VEGF helps prevent further growth of the blood vessels that the cancer needs to continue growing." Again the 'C' word! I couldn't handle this stress! My body started to pump more and more adrenaline into my system. I could have shot through the roof from all of it storing inside of me. All I needed was an ejection button on the side of my chair and away I would go.

She continued reading, "The goal of treatment is to prevent further loss of vision." She explained that they would numb my eye with multiple drops and then Dr. Stewart would do the injection in the top portion of my eye. This was going to have to be done every four to six weeks until the blood vessel decided to stop rupturing. And then, to end my nice doomsday consent, she finished with

Clarity

listing the possible complications from the medication. Some complications for patients who were being treated for cancer were "gastrointestinal perforations or wound healing complications, hemorrhage, stroke, heart attack, hypertension, proteinuria, and congestive heart failure." Cancer patients were given "400 times the dose" that I would be given, but this information still didn't sit well with me regardless of that fact. Then she continued to list out the complications for the eye, which was completely a separate list than the one given previously.

The handout stated that complications were low, but the FDA didn't actually approve the use of this medication for the purpose of eye injections. The nurse continued reading that the medication may help my condition, but it wasn't, for sure, going to help it get better. Lastly, I could have an allergic reaction to the medication if I have other allergies or if I have asthma, which I had both currently. "Symptoms of an allergic reaction can include a rash, hives, itching, shortness of breath, and rarely death." I could also experience other issues with my eye like "cataracts, glaucoma, retinal detachment, pressure issues, possible eye infections, floaters, eye pain, and swelling."[2]

I sat their numb. She handed me the pen and paper to sign, and I couldn't do it. I froze like a deer in headlights. Gary had already taken the kids back to the waiting room. I so wished he had been there to help me mentally go through everything she just read. I stumbled on my words from tears choking my throat. I finally got out some sound and said, "This is really scary. Everything you just read doesn't sound good at all. Cancer medication, possible stroke, infections... I don't know." She pushed back with urgency, not allowing me to feel the real repercussions of the decision I was about to make. I reluctantly signed the paperwork and prayed that I would be okay.

Immediately, they started putting numbing drops in my eye and preparing me for the invasion of my eyeball. The room started to fill up with staff that earlier I agreed to let watch this brave attempt to save my sight. My anxiety came to an all-time high as Dr. Stewart walked in with his head covered with a surgeon's cap and a face mask. In my mind, I thought, *Help, this is happening... he's prepped and ready to go. This is serious. Oh my God! I can't do this!*

He leaned me back in the cushioned chair and I stared up at the ceiling as the staff of about six all stared at me. His voice was calm and I found some comfort in hearing him explain everything that he was going to do. My breathing was erratic and my hands were clammy. I had to do this, I didn't have a choice, but every part of my being wanted to run. Dr. Stewart placed a round, cold, metal clamp around my eye to hold my eyelids open. He placed a few more numbing drops in my eyes, and told me to look down and to my left shoulder. His words, "light pinch" still ring in my ears. It was a strange sensation of the needle entering into my eye. It was quick and a pinch just like he said. They removed the eye clamp, and, suddenly, after rinsing my eye with some solution, my throat started to feel like it was closing up. I couldn't swallow and the panic started to set in.

I quickly tried to get the word out to let them know something was wrong. Immediately, they started asking me questions and I couldn't talk. My throat was squeezing and my breathing was fast. I started to literally shake. My whole body was trembling like I was shivering cold. Yet I wasn't freezing at all, I was sweating and scared. *Crap,* I thought, *is this it? Is this how I die? Is my eye really what takes me out?* My husband's and babies' faces flashed in my mind. They were sitting in the waiting room and had no idea what was happening to me. This couldn't be it! I had a family I had to be there for.

In a blurred moment, the staff started to work around me in a swift like motion. Someone handed me water to try to drink, another person brought in an oxygen tank and attached the mask to my face, another stood by with an EpiPen, waiting for the doctor's orders, the doctor was listening to my lungs with a cold stethoscope, and the other staff members were staring at me with wide, worried eyes. I heard my doctor's voice switch from authoritative to calm, "Your airways are still open. How is your throat?" I took another sip of water and finally it started to relax. I choked out that it was better. The nurse asked if I felt cold. I responded "No" in a confused voice until I realized that I was still shaking. I found my voice enough to

Clarity

finally explain that I had the same shaking reaction when I had epidurals with my three children. Each time I was given one, the shaking was worse. I asked what the numbing drops were and it was Lidocaine with Epinephrine. The doctor was pretty confident that I had an adrenaline dump/panic attack. I, on the other hand, wasn't so sure what had just happened. In my gut there was more to it than just me being scared, but I was exhausted at this point, so I didn't press the issue any more.

    The nurse stayed with me for what seemed like an hour while I breathed in the oxygen. I finally stopped shaking and my husband and kids were able to come in and see me. I had never felt so relieved to see them. I hugged them so tight and promised myself that I would figure this out. I couldn't do this again. We slowly made our way out to the waiting room and rescheduled my next appointment for four weeks at the same clinic. The pain in my eye was intense on the way home and I struggled to open it. My body felt like it was just hit by a train. All of my muscles were sore from tensing up and shaking, and my head hurt from the crying and from the intense stress. I was a hot mess once again.

    A few days went by and life felt like torture. My eye felt like someone had punched me directly in the eye socket. It ached so much once we got home that I called Dr. Redman that evening to ask if that was supposed to happen. He was concerned and had me come in the next day to take a look at everything. After taking a look, he said everything looked good, but it was going to take some time to adjust to the medication being in my eye. He was absolutely right! The medication was moving the fluid so much that, at one point, I couldn't drive my truck anymore. My eyes were not only fighting with each other for a perfect image, but now I was also seeing distorted images. A section of my vision in my right eye made everything appear like it was going in and coming out of a portal tube. The motion of cars driving around me made the images even worse. What I was viewing looked so futuristic as the vehicle would turn into a wavy, opaque, slime-looking tube I was seeing and stretch out until it popped out of the other side of the tube. I felt as though I was seeing something from a strange alien movie.

I went back again to see Dr. Redman and asked for an eye patch. I couldn't use both of my eyes at the same time. I couldn't wear contacts and my glasses weren't any help either. I suddenly felt like I was already blind. What good were my eyes if I couldn't even use them? I felt lost in a sea of emotions. I was extremely embarrassed and scared about what this meant for my future. My vision was worse now than what it was before I went to Dr. Stewart. A flashback of my chiropractic experience came into my head. Did I just ignore my voice again, and now I'm in an even worse position? I was so torn on how I felt about this. I really didn't have a choice in the moment of what to do for my eye, but I couldn't shake the feeling that I was on a downward spiral of constant health misery.

I came home from teaching at our martial arts school one evening feeling exhausted and distraught and I pulled out my patch. Looking down at it, I thought about how I had struggled all day with being there. My eyes were making me nauseous because they were working so hard to see an image clearly together. My right eye was my dominant eye, which meant I had to now try and get my left eye to do the heavy lifting. It was as if my eyes were at war with each other. The right eye was damaged, but didn't want to give up power to the left eye. This constant strain left me with headaches and a feeling in my eye socket like I had just gotten punched by Muhammad Ali. I twirled the black, silk like patch in my hands. My eyes watered and an idea came to my head.

I had seen a book back in my college days at a local bookstore. I didn't buy the book, but I intently looked at the pictures and had gotten a good glimpse of what the book was about. A Japanese scientist did a study about water and how it takes on positive or negative words and mimics them. In college, I had the thought about healing the body using words and how useful that would be since the body is made up of mostly water. I twirled the patch again and as I studied it, the more I realized I had to put a word on my patch. I couldn't write a positive word on my eyelid, out of fear of embarrassment and infections. But, I could write a word on my eye patch. I had a choice in this moment. Was I going to let this disease beat me or was I going to beat it.

Clarity

I looked at my children playing and my husband cooking dinner. I had to write something powerful, and it had to mean something more than just healing. It had to be impactful and something that I wanted out of this whole experience. I didn't want to be the girl who just rolled over and drowned in mystery. So the word came to me... *Clarity!* I then realized what I wanted. I needed to find Clarity in this whole process. That was what I was searching for. I needed clarity on why this happened and what this whole horrible situation was trying to teach me. There had to be a reason. It couldn't just be a disease; I wouldn't accept that.

Luckily, my kids and I loved to do art projects. I quickly dug through some supplies and I found the cutest clear gemstones. I started to stick one of them onto the patch and realized it wasn't going to adhere to the silky fabric. I got up and found some super glue. As my husband watched from the kitchen, I attempted to put a drop of glue on the gem and stick it on the patch. My eyes were playing tricks on me, and I couldn't align the super glue dropper to the small gem I held so carefully. I tried a few times and finally the frustration put me into full blown tears. Crocodile-sized tears steadily rolled down my face as I literally hung my head in defeat.

My sweet husband turned his back on the halfway cooked dinner and came over to the table where I was sitting. He put his sympathetic hand on my back ever so gently, held me close to him, and asked what was wrong. I bit through my tears and explained to him that I just wanted to write Clarity on this stupid patch, but I couldn't do it because I couldn't line up the glue to the gem. He said, "I got this. It's okay." He slowly put his manly, supporting hand on mine and took the glue out of my hand. He pulled up a chair and started to glue the gems on one-by-one until it formed the word Clarity.

As I sat there and watched him take such pride in helping me, I realized in this moment that we both had made a choice. We made a choice together, without saying it out loud, that we were going to do whatever it took to get me back to my normal self again. I saw the worry and the scared look on his face when he sat there looking at the patch. It was uncertainty and fearfulness of the future. Neither of us knew what the future held for us, but we both knew that we couldn't do it alone. I fell more in love with my husband that day than any other day. In that moment, I realized that he would do anything for me, no matter how silly it seemed, to help me heal to my full self. That word *Clarity* took on a whole new meaning for the both of us, and we were determined to find the true meaning of this horrible situation that I was in.

Part 2

In this section of the book, you'll be following along with my story to better understand what I did to heal. You'll also learn how it can help you on your journey. As I tell my story, you will also be introduced to where you can find out more information or how this can and will apply to your life and your healing journey. I want to encourage you to take notes, follow along, and, in each section, start to ask yourself how does or could this apply to you. Everyone has a story. Some people yell their story out, and others keep their story stuck inside of them where it festers like a nasty virus.

I only ask one thing as you go through this book: don't keep your story away from your healing. Your story is important and it explains the reasons why your situation exists today. As you read through the chapters, think about your story and listen to the voice you hear inside of you. Maybe it doesn't sound all that strong, or maybe you were like me where Superwoman wanted to come out and tackle every situation; either way, hear it and work with it. Use the activities and steps in the next section to help you figure out how you got in the situation you're in, and how you can get out of it. As you interact with the story, allow your inner self to lead you to a path of healing and discovery.

Chapter 2: Saying "Enough"

    The next few weeks were mentally and physically draining. I saw Dr. Stewart a few weeks later. He had great news that the fluid in my eye didn't appear to be coming back. Even though my eye was still adjusting to all of the newness, I was able to leave the clinic without an injection that day. Suddenly my good news vanished a week later when my vision took a rapid turn for the worse. I ended up in an emergency visit with Dr. Stewart again. This time it was in a different office that was closer to home. As we drove to Rhinelander, Wisconsin, I couldn't breathe. My vision had catapulted backward so quickly in a week's time. I could feel my eye swelling in the back and my warped vision showed a problem was rapidly occurring again. Straight lined objects were replaced with wavy lines making it look as though I was in a circus fun house.

    We pulled up to a small, older looking building. It was quite different than the one we had been to before. I felt a weird peace come over me with the notion that this place wasn't so enormous and overwhelming. My squeezing throat experience didn't sit well with me from that last visit in the large, unpredictable building. I didn't want to repeat that event, so I welcomed anything new to my already shaky environment. This older, well-maintained building wasn't as nice as the fancy building in Wausau, but it made me feel like I was someone. I wasn't going to just get shuffled among all the other gobs of people. This place weirdly brought me comfort and hope. Little did I know, this building was going to hold my transformational struggles and successes.

    I walked into the building and was immediately rerouted to the basement level. Feeling apprehensive, I still tried to hang onto

Clarity

the fact that this place was better. We made our way to the waiting room where smells of old wallpaper and mildew struck my nose. I turned right into the windowless waiting room and was reminded how much I didn't belong in this situation. All of these wonderful, elderly eyes looked at me suddenly with question marks on their brows. I hung my head as I walked to my seat through the crowd of about 10 people who were in their 70s or older, feeling exposed, embarrassed, and defeated.

After getting called back to the exam room, my fear was now becoming a reality as the young, studious looking doctor entered the room behind me. My eye was still in a volcanic eruption and was threatening to take my beloved sight. I started to panic as he expressed the need for another injection. I gripped my throat as I asked the question, "What if I have a reaction again?" He calmly and confidently reassured me that I would be okay and they had a hunch it was the epinephrine in the lidocaine that caused the reaction. He replied again with confidence and suggested using a different way to numb my eye. Reluctantly, I agreed and the procedure started again. This time was with fewer people and a lot more sympathy for my already shocked system. Luckily, the procedure went much better. That unfortunately didn't stop the physical pain in my eye and my emotional pain in my heart that were still pulsating at an intense level.

I suddenly had a new life thrown on me. What I thought would be a one-time fix turned into a constant real nightmare. I had a whole slew of health problems at this point, and things weren't looking up. My back and right side were still in pain from some unknown source, my nerves were still being tickled by slow torture, and my stomach couldn't handle food without blowing up to feel and look like I was carrying a small baby elephant. To add to all of that, now my right eye had decided to start a small volcanic leak deep within. According to Dr. Stewart, it didn't look like there was an end in sight. No pun intended. To make the situation worse, my family doctor ran blood labs to see if anything showed up there, and, of course, they came up empty handed. Between my family doctor, chiropractor, physical therapist, and my eye doctors, none of them had any answers as to why my health had deteriorated so rapidly.

Emotionally I was in turmoil. I could hold things together for the outside world to see, but inside I was mixed with anger, resentment, frustration, and hate; pretty much every negative emotion you could think of filled me up. My patch had become something that I relied on each day for various things. Sometimes I had to wear it driving (when I absolutely had to drive), at times I wore it at home just to give my eyes a break from working so hard, and most of the time I had to wear it while I tried to look at the computer screen to do my busy paperwork for our never-ending businesses. Time didn't stop for anyone, and so I had to use this patch to help me shuffle along my new life.

Since my doctors didn't have a whole lot of answers for me as to what I was experiencing with this uneven, warped vision, I decided to wear the patch whenever I felt like I needed to. I looked at it daily, asking for clarity. It was the one word that I hung onto. I decided to fix my eye because not fixing it hurt more than the condition itself. As the days went on and my depression grew worse and more deeply rooted, I kept reminding myself that this brick wall that I faced wasn't the answer. I had to find clarity! If I didn't, I would end up on an even faster spiral downward. I couldn't let my children or my husband see me like that.

I knew my answers weren't going to just show up at my doorstep as a nicely wrapped present. Nope, I had to do the work to figure this out. I struggled with my gumption to pull myself together, but over a few weeks, I started to research my condition to save myself and to save the perception my kids had of me. To my amazement, my shy bravery to find the answers resulted in nothing! I showed up, I started to research, and then I honestly couldn't find any valuable information other than what my doctors already had given me. "Really?!" I yelled out loud. How was it possible that in our day and age, there wasn't anything other than the information on what happens in the eye and this crazy cancer medication that wasn't even intended for the eye. I shook my head in frustration as I realized my search had ended in a matter of a few hours. I called my sister, Malina, and cried on the phone. I asked her for advice and she simply said "Nik, I think you just have to accept that this is your new normal." I hung up the phone, and just dropped in tears from the reality of her statement. "No! This isn't okay! I have had ENOUGH!" I silently yelled to myself so I wouldn't disturb my kids. I had to find another way.

WHAT I DID AND WHAT YOU CAN DO: ACTION STEPS 1-4

> **Find Another Way:**

I couldn't find the research supporting the condition I had, but I could find loads of information on a disease close to it called Macular Degeneration. I used this as my framework to understand the eye and what it was doing. I also started to research the medication I was on. I became a student in this disease. I knew that, to my doctors, I was just another case, another patient who needed an injection. They weren't going to be dedicated to me and my personal decision to heal this, once and for all, like I wish they could be. It was up to me, and it's up to you to figure out what will help you heal.

> **Step 1 - Make a Decision:**

In order to heal, you first have to start with the mindset that you want to heal. How badly do you want your condition to change? What's your WHY? You have to determine why you want to heal, and that will help you focus all of your energy on the tasks at hand. If you're why isn't strong enough, you'll fall victim to settling. When it comes to your health, DON'T settle. Do whatever it takes to get yourself back to a healthy state. Remember all of the things worth fighting for, and if it helps, make a list of the things that support your why.

It all starts with a mind shift in the right direction. This can be difficult to navigate through, since your emotions are fighting negativity. But even a small glimmer of possibility can catapult you to a better you. It all starts with a positive thought of "I can change this." My guess is, since you're reading this book, you've already made the first step to a better you. Way to go! Now roll up those sleeves and let's dig into getting you closer to your WHY.

> **Step 2 - Do the Research Yourself:**

Don't take what you hear from the doctors as absolute truth. Your doctors are doing the best job they can with your condition. And don't get me wrong, they do have more schooling under their belt than either of us have. Heck, they know this disease at this point better than you do. But, they don't know your body and your mind the way you do. And, they don't know the trauma or stress you have/had in your life. They care about you, but nobody will care as much as you do about your health. The better you understand the problem, the better you can see the solution. I encourage you to get down and dirty with your progress. Research all that you can about your condition. Explore things that are closely connected, and stretch your mind on avenues that doctors won't explore in depth, like possibly your stress levels. I will get into more examples of this as you continue.

If you get stuck on finding the information that you're looking for, ask a family member to help you. Sometimes, a person who isn't experiencing the actual disease will have a different way of looking up the information. Since they aren't attached to it the way you are, it will be less emotionally draining for them to navigate through the information.

However, don't forget that an important part of healing is listening to that inner voice. Sometimes, you might come across some information, and as you read it, that little voice speaks up and says, "OHHH YES, THAT'S ME; I have that!" This is important to tap into and write down. It's a very good possibility that you found a clue to your healing progress.

As you move through this research portion of your healing, allow yourself time to digest what you've read as well. Don't get bogged down with the negativity outcomes that might be listed on websites, books, or articles you read; rather, keep focusing on the process of why it happens in the body as an overall picture. Sometimes, seeing diagrams or watching videos on what the disease process looks like, will help you understand the dis-ease in your body better. This knowledge can help you ask more questions or start to put the pieces together in a more logical way, instead of the panic notion of scrambled woe's-me thoughts.

Clarity

You might have noticed above that I spelled disease as dis-ease. Yes, dis-ease. Your body is at a point that it is not at ease within itself. Your job, detective, is to find the answers to put your body back into a balanced state of ease. Your job is not to dwell on the spiraling staircase that some have laid out for you. You're strong and will find the research you need. As you go through the process, keep focusing on finding ease, and that the scary word *disease* is something you can break apart and change into ease again. It's all about mindset.

> **Step 3 - Work with your Doctor:**

Yes, although I stated to do your own research, that doesn't mean to ignore your doctor's advice. You'll need to find a balance of listening to your inner voice, while also hearing and working with your doctor's advice. They aren't the enemy if they don't have all the answers. Or maybe your doctor is the kind of person who thinks he has all the answers and wants to shove them down your throat. Either way, it's your job to hear them, take their advice into consideration, and make your own choices along the way.

Make sure that you talk to your doctors about the research you discovered in Step 2. They should know you're digging deep and they most likely will help you uncover hidden hints for future research. Your doctor will also help you understand the medical jargon you find in your research. So please, work with them and allow them to help you become a successful detective in your own case. If by chance they wave a hand at you and are unsupportive in your research, do it anyways, and maybe look for a more supportive doctor. I'm passing a little superhero power to you in this moment to PROVE THEM WRONG, and show them you can heal. (Superwoman and I are friends now.) This will empower you to find the answers and heal. It's your wonderful body and life, and you deserve to heal, so move mountains!

> **Step 4 - Document Everything:**

One of the best ways you can keep track of your progress is to document everything that you find important. I started a binder to keep my information within. As I learned more about my eye, I wanted to look back and see my progress. Within my binder, I held the medication consent form, images of my OCT scans of the inner eye, lab results, home water test results, food related issues, documents that I found helpful, websites that I wanted to look into more, etc. You can add anything in this binder related to your questions, thoughts, or research. I also brought this binder to each appointment that I had. I wanted my doctors to understand how serious I was about fixing this problem, and the binder created legs for me to stand on when asking them questions about my condition. Having all of your information in one place is also a way to keep yourself grounded. For myself, I often flipped through all the information to grab motivation to keep going or to reward myself on the success I had along the way. This step is super important and is a must do in your healing journey!

** YOUR TO-DO LIST **

1. WRITE DOWN YOUR DECISION AND SPECIFY YOUR WHY IN YOUR BINDER.
2. START RESEARCHING EVERYTHING YOU CAN ABOUT YOUR SITUATION.
3. ASK YOUR DOCTORS THE HARD QUESTIONS, BUT WORK WITH THEM.
4. BUY A BINDER AND DOCUMENT ALL YOUR FINDINGS.

Chapter 3: Connecting the Dots

After hearing my sister's words, I realized how hard this was going to be. I talked to my husband more in depth that night and expressed to him my struggles. He looked at me and simply asked, "What's your WHY?" I looked confused at him, wondering what the heck he was talking about. He was brilliant at business and I figured he would have something to say that would relate back to his training. He continued, "You know this isn't going to be easy, but you have to know why you're doing something. If you know why you're doing it, then the steps to get there will become easier to see. So, what's your why?" I looked at him and tears flooded my eyes. I knew the answer to his question, but it hurt to say it. I finally choked out with big raindrop tears running down my cheeks, "My why is to make sure I can see my kids' faces as they grow up."

Oh, did it hit me like a punch to the gut as I said the words. Saying it made it more real, and I knew, in that moment, that I wasn't going to stop searching for the answer. How could I? I had three amazingly beautiful little children who had a lifetime ahead of them. I didn't want to miss that! My husband was right; my why was strong enough to fight through the difficulties I was about to face. Without answers to the problem, I was going to have to find them no matter what, and I had to rely on my WHY to motivate me through the thick mess.

The next few weeks, I worked with my depression alongside finding research articles. I had to work with my grief, but I couldn't let myself be consumed by it. I had to stay focused on the end goal of saving my sight when the doctors told me I was at high risk for blindness. Although my depression was pulling on me, my husband always found suggestions to help me through all the tears. Although his silly humor always made me laugh, he also suggested we watch *Game of Thrones*. To go along with the show, my new title these days was Patch Wearing, Fitness Instructor, The Mother of an Emotional Mess, Slayer of Ice Cream Cartons. I was fixated on this show of misery and death, yet surprisingly, watching this and letting myself go through the grieving stages gave me confidence. My life wasn't that bad after watching this mystical land's problems. I found strength that these people, although they were made up, would keep going and keep fighting no matter what. I found the power to say, "I am powerful, and I can do this!"

Now that I found some magical power from within, I started to connect the dots. I had a gut feeling that all of my health problems at the time were all connected to my eye. Although all of my doctors combined thought it was a shot in the dark, the nagging thought of fixing this wouldn't leave me. I decided to play with ideas I had running through my head and I started back at the beginning. It didn't take me long to remember the first symptoms I had were my food baby stomach, and the side/back pain. How could that be connected to my eye? It would be an angle the doctors wouldn't think of, and it was possible there could be a connection.

I started looking up macular degeneration, since that was closely related to my condition and there was loads more information on that than choroidal neovascular membrane. One search brought me to a website by Dr. Joshua Axe that changed the game for me. In an article, listed on his site written by Jillian Levy, CHHC, she talked about what kind of diet to be on and what types of things could cause issues like this to begin with.[3] Finally! I found a connection. It wasn't much, but my hope started to bubble up deep within me. I started to feel a buzzing vibration from the hope, and I realized I found a glimmer of possibility in all the darkness.

Digging into the article, I realized just how many people had to deal with the same fate that I was dealing with. Levy continued with her information about macular degeneration by stating, "That means 196 million adults worldwide will have at least partially lost their vision due to this disorder by 2020 and an estimated 288 million by 2040."[3] Suddenly, I didn't feel so alone. This disease

Clarity

wasn't out to just get me; it was after a lot of people. Could there be a connection to all of us?

Reading on, I started to sift through the information about diets. I realized that I wasn't eating enough veggies and fruits that would support my eye. I also wasn't taking any vitamins to help with the process either. I wasn't a smoker or a drinker, so those recommendations didn't apply to me, but I was eating quite a bit of sugar. I had to retire my Slayer of Ice Cream Cartons title and quickly. As a fitness instructor, I knew that part wasn't healthy for me, but grief had taken over. Now it was time for me to take the power back from grief.

My curiosities on food led me to keep searching Dr. Axe's website. I wanted to figure out why my stomach kept reacting to foods, and maybe if I focused on that, I would at least heal one part of my body. My search led me to learn more about leaky gut. I quickly signed up for a webinar that explained what it was. I didn't know anything about this term, but I was grabbing onto any clues I could that would help me heal.

The night of the webinar, I was buzzing around the house before it started. My husband had noticed my excitement and asked what was happening. He was used to seeing me crying and sulking, so this bubbly person seemed unfamiliar to him. I quickly explained and jumped on the webinar without letting him get a word in. The information that was delivered was incredible. I suddenly went from not knowing what leaky gut was to understanding that I had all of the symptoms for it. (See the next section for more information regarding leaky gut.) The biggest symptom that I had was food sensitivity. I quickly learned that this could be contributing to my chronic fatigue, my issues with food, and my pain. I also had other issues in the past like asthma and IBS that could also be from developing leaky gut syndrome. I was weirdly thrilled to learn these too could also be linked to my overall condition.

I enrolled in Dr. Axe's Leaky Gut Program and took his online Leaky Gut Test. After getting the quick results back, I realized that I was testing 100% for two of the five "gut types." The five groups listed were "Stressed Gut, Candida Gut, Immune Gut,

Gastric Gut, and Gallbladder Gut."[4-8] The two groups that were elevated for me was Candida and Immune Gut.

I sat back and said out loud, "Wow! I really do have some serious issues!" My husband stopped his sarcastic giggle when he realized I wasn't joking and my demeanor was all business. My mind was exploding with information about these two different leaky gut types and all the dots started to align. I started to check the boxes off for my symptoms: Chronic Fatigue?... check, Mood Disorders?... check, Urinary Tract Infections?... uncheck, Oral Thrush?... check, Sinus Infections?... uncheck, Intestinal Distress?... big check, Brain Fog?... Check, Skin and Nail Infections?... uncheck, Hormonal Imbalance?... check. This list also mentioned high amounts of stress and grief could also contribute to the issues. Those two words held a heavy burden on me.

Here it was all laid out for me. I started to go through the food lists and compiled a list of different foods to eat and not to eat in order to heal the intestinal lining. I finally felt like I had a plan to take me to the next path in healing my eye. My overall assumption was that if I wasn't absorbing the proper minerals and vitamins from my intestines, how could my eye get what it needed to heal. I started to process even further. What if the stress and grief I had felt for so long led my body to break down in my gut first. I excitedly realized that, without the proper absorption and also toxins potentially going through my intestinal lining, somehow this would travel up and affect my eye in a negative way. Could it be that my system just needed to heal in my stomach in order for my eye to heal? I was willing to give it a shot. At this point, I didn't have any other options. This foundation was extremely important to help support me through the crazy ride that I was about to take.

WHAT I DID AND WHAT YOU CAN DO: ACTION STEPS 5-8

> **Connecting the Dots:**

A note on Leaky Gut: According to Marcelo Campos, MD from Harvard Health Publishing/Harvard Medical School "An unhealthy gut lining may have large cracks or holes, allowing partially digested food, toxins, and bugs to penetrate the tissues beneath it. This may trigger inflammation and changes in the gut flora (normal bacteria) that could lead to problems within the digestive tract and beyond."[9] Although I used Dr. Axes program to help launch me into my first steps of healing, I stayed open to any other websites or research articles that came my way. For the purpose of this book, I will mostly stick to the information that Dr. Axe gives on his website because I found it extremely credible, laid out in an easy manner to understand, and it gave easy steps to get better. I would highly recommend taking a look at his site and doing a search for your condition underneath him. You can find links to his site by visiting www.nikkiengels.com/draxe to learn more..

> ➢ **Step 5 - Follow Your Grief:**

Grief is an interesting animal. It can keep you down, or, at a moment's notice, it can shift and push you into a wild monster with emotions spewing out of you. For me, I had to just go through the stages and let myself really feel all of the emotions as they came to me. According to Healgrief.org, the five stages are

- "Denial: This can't be happening.
- Anger: Why did this happen? Who is to blame?
- Bargaining: Make this not happen and I will…
- Depression: I can't bear this; I'm too sad to do anything
- Acceptance: I acknowledge that this has happened and I cannot change it.

Although these stages are presented in a neat and concise format, there's nothing neat or concise when it comes to one's personal journey with grief."[10]

Now that you can see clearly how grief is laid out, you also have to give it room to do what it wants. What does that mean for you? Feel it, let it out in a scream, and breathe through all areas of it. You need to give yourself forgiveness for feeling all the emotions that you are. Each of these stages presents themselves very differently in all of us, and you need to follow your body's lead through that. Your body is an amazing temple, and if it needs to let out a frustrating scream, it's your job to let it do that.

Think of it this way, it's your body's way of getting rid of negative energy. Thus, treat your body like a temple. So many people often get swept up in the depression of things and get lost along the way. While you're following your grief, do whatever you can to help your body heal, and work through all of those stages. Things like alcohol, drugs, or any other substance abuse aren't the answer. Stick with ice cream. It's a lot easier to cut out once you come out on the other side. If you're battling with your grief and have dabbled with substance use of some kind, this is your time to find the help you need, and get the support system that your body is craving for.

Eventually, you'll get through this obstacle you're facing, but remember, make it easy on your system. Your body needs and deserves you to fight for its health, happiness, and love. Immerse yourself with good, nonthreatening ways to find your motivation and inspiration. A few ideas you can put forth is watch a funny movie every night, read a book that makes you feel like a bad-ass, take a kickboxing class to work out your frustrations, or maybe carve out some time to travel with your loved ones.

> **Step 6 - Have a Cheerleader and Inspiration:**

This step is extremely important. You will most likely face obstacles throughout your healing journey. Although that sounds scary, learn to embrace it, but also have someone to help hold you up. Your task throughout this part is to find someone to really express yourself to. It can be your spouse, a sibling, another family member, best friend, etc.

Your cheerleader has to follow these guidelines:
- ★ They must really listen to you.
  - They must take the time to give you their undivided attention. No cell phones, no distraction. They're truly there to hear your success and struggles with healing.
- ★ They are your rock.
  - When times are tough, this person is there to help you keep going. They are that little voice that tells you, "YOU got this!" You'll need to be reminded often that you're

doing the right thing. Expect that your doctors will tell you, "Things looks slim." This person, however, never says that to you. They're steady and true to your success.
- ★ They keep it light.
  - ○ Laughter is the best medicine. This person should be able to find the humor in the situation and allow you to feel and laugh about the crazy journey. They respectfully know how to get a smile on your face. Or they know when they need to break out *Game of Thrones* to bring you back to being a brave queen/king.
- ★ They are supportive no matter what.
  - ○ They are the person that you know you can call whenever you need them, day or night. If you need to bounce an idea off of them, they'll help you dig for research. If you're really happy, they should put on some music and dance with you. If you're really sad, they should know how to pick your mood up without crying themselves.

If you find yourself reading this step and are scratching your head saying, "Well what about me? I don't have that person. Can my dog be that person?" Well, although your dog or other pet will help you with the healing journey, you're really going to need to have a physical person who can talk and tell you when you need to calm down. At times, you'll need someone to shake you and bring you back to reality. You'll need a person to help you push this imaginary boulder up the mountain. A dog can be there for snuggles but is useless when it comes to the shaking and pushing factor. If you need to find a support buddy, visit www.nikkiengels.com/groups to chat with others who are on their healing journey.

> **Step 7 - Connect Your Dots:**
I often talk about getting dirty and digging deep. You have to do this step to get to the root cause of what's happening to you. I said it earlier, and I'll say it again, ONLY YOU know what got you here. Other people can give you glimmers of realization, but you're the only one that can hear your thoughts, hurts, and biggest desires. This is your time to hear yourself and put it all on paper. Your step

for this section is to create a spider web of ideas. I'm going to reference the inner superhero in you and trust that your thoughts will link together like the strings of a spider web. We'll call this your HEALING WEB. Please visit www.nikkiengels.com/downloads to find the Healing Web for you to make copies of and start listing your ideas.

In your web, start with your condition in the middle. On the outer lines start listing out all the symptoms that you feel are connected. There's no right or wrong way to do this, so dump all your ideas, feelings, and gut intuitions on this paper. Once you feel like you have everything on your Healing Web, pick out the very first thing that you think happened to you on this web. This is your first clue and a place to start. Now, put your healing web in your binder. You don't have to look at this every day, but use it as a reference when something comes up. Also feel free to jot down notes or new ideas that come to you as you move forward in this book.

➢ **Step 8 - Take Consistent Action:**

You might have heard a story some time in your life about pushing an imaginary boulder up a hill, relating to how hard it is to obtain success. For a better visual, I'm going to change the story. Let's use a ridiculous image of me, Patch Wearing, Fitness Instructor, Mother of an Emotional Mess, Slayer of Ice Cream Cartons, rolling a large, oversized eyeball up a mountain. A little creepy, I know, but stay with me.

In order to save my sight in this eyeball, I have to get it all the way to the top of the mountain to a medicine man. This man has all the answers that I need and a sacred holistic approach to heal my eye. I get a fourth of the way up, muck hits my feet, I'm tired, and I don't feel like I can hold the weight of this swollen eyeball. I know if I let go, it will crush me underneath the size of it. I'm tired and don't know where to turn. I call out to my little leprechaun in my shirt pocket. I say, "Eager McNoodles, I need your luck! I can't do this anymore! The muck is too thick and I'm drowning in misery holding the weight of this enormous eyeball. What do I do?" He answers back in a squeaky but authoritative voice, "Remember your why, my friend, and let it lead you to the top. You'll find strength there." He slowly slides back into my pocket to wait for his chance to again share his luck and good fortune. I decide to keep going, since Eager McNoodles was right. My why would help lead me a little bit at a time. I just had to focus on it.

I feel the traction starting to build in my body to reach the top when I finally reach the halfway point. I smile inside as I stood on Success Ledge. I take a breath and celebrate my success with a happy leprechaun dance. Continuing on, I eventually reach the last 10 feet of Healed Mountain where Medicine Man awaits. He greets me in his colorful robes of beauty, and is happy to help push the eyeball the rest of the way. Medicine Man looks at me and says, "You've proven to me and to yourself how badly you wanted to succeed. I am happy to join you on your journey and allow you to see the gift of Healed Mountain. The gift will be revealed in time."

Yes, a ridiculous story, but I bet you won't forget it! As you travel along your journey, remind yourself of the mountain that you're on. You have to do the hard work! If you don't do it, what does life look like? Probably not what you really want, right?! So what does that mean? It means that every day you dig in and research a little more. You eat a meal that day that's more nutritious than the day before, and you find something happy from your day and you focus on that instead of all the drama and stress that might surround you.

Your task is to find the golden nuggets and reach your Success Ledge. Start to imagine yourself finding the answers and you taking a breath on Success Ledge. Gathering your strength and carry on, inching higher a little each day. Doing this over and over again will start to create the feeling inside your heart that you can reach the top. Your adventure journey is Healed Mountain and you now have 8 tools (steps) in your pocket to lead the way! Once you're finally healed, you'll look back and realize the journey was the gift and you've been transformed into a stronger and better person.

** YOUR TO-DO LIST **
5. LET YOUR GRIEF BREATH THE WAY IT NEEDS TO.
6. MAKE A MENTAL NOTE OF WHO YOUR CHEERLEADER IS.
7. FILL OUT YOUR HEALING WEB.
8. KEEP MOVING FORWARD EVERY DAY. LITTLE THINGS ADD UP TO BIG THINGS!

Clarity

Chapter 4: Gut Health

It is now five months since I was diagnosed with this rare eye disease. I've already had five injections up to this point. The medication was working to stop the growth of the blood vessel and was allowing time for my eye to reabsorb the fluid. However, I was still struggling with my sight. The inner eye still had a lot of swelling and I was now building up scar tissue. This didn't help with the discrepancies between my two eyes. I had to repeatedly go into my local eye doctors to adjust my glasses to create a symmetric image. I kept complaining that my eyes were not working together and I felt a horrible pulling sensation between them. My headaches were becoming more intense and I just felt sick to my stomach from trying to put together a clear image.

Dr. Stewart stayed pretty firm on the fact that reducing stress and changing my food habits wouldn't really help in this situation. Although, occasionally, he would give a glimmer of hope that this blood vessel could burn itself out and be done. He continued that some people only needed a few shots and others would need shots for the rest of their lives. This was an odd statement, since most of his clients were already in their 70s. That's a very different approach to look at when your doctor says that and you're only 32. I tried to find comfort in the idea that this could just abruptly end, but, unfortunately, my scans didn't show that was going to happen any time soon. I was pushing my appointments out for injections to every six weeks. By the time I would go back to see Dr. Stewart for the next appointment, the massive black hole was back, threatening to take my sight. After an injection, the hole like shape would settle back down, and I would also feel a relief from the pressure building in the back of the eye.

It was a blessing that I even had this option to begin with. I knew in my heart that had this not been a treatment option, I would have already lost the battle. These shots were giving me the time I needed to figure out the root cause of this. I knew that the medication was only a band aid, but my body couldn't keep up with the effects they had on me. With each injection, I would become so tired that I would sleep for hours afterwards. My skin suddenly wasn't healing if I broke out with acne, and I felt like I had cold-like symptoms for days afterwards with flashes of hot and cold chills. I was also still dealing with the nerve pain as well. I felt as though my body was deteriorating before me.

I kept searching for the answers my eye desperately needed by studying the issues I had with my stomach. I learned all I could about gut health and leaky gut issues. I also started to switch all of my food products, make-up, and body care products all to organic and plant based. I had learned that products that were filled with chemicals and GMOs were putting my system into more distress. I couldn't afford to put anything in my body at this point that wasn't pure and wholesome. It was a big decision for our family to put organic products first. I had to relearn how to shop all over again, because, unfortunately, it was quite a bit more expensive.

I also started a food journal of what foods were bothering my stomach. I could tell within a few minutes if something agreed with me or not. The reaction my stomach would have to food was so immediate that even my family could tell when it happened. There was no denying the elephant baby stomach that would immediately pop up. Before going organic, every food seemed to do it. As I switched over to eating cleaner, I was able to more accurately put in the journal which foods bothered my system. I had narrowed the big irritants down to wheat, eggs, corn or corn starch, dairy, pork, and sugar. Once I figured these items were causing issues, I took them out of my diet immediately.

Using Dr. Axe's guidelines to help heal the stomach with various foods and taking out the irritants, my stomach started to feel better and had fewer reactions. My diet was pretty simple. It consisted of chicken; turkey; bone broth; sauerkraut; cooked veggies like kale, onions, squash, spinach, carrots, cauliflower, celery, and asparagus; fresh fruit like blueberries and green apples; quinoa; coconut oil; avocados; coconut flour; spices like ginger and turmeric; flaxseeds; and lots of pure water, especially lemon water. This was a hard adjustment for my whole family. We were now cooking meals completely different than before. I was amazed at how much my family supported me on this journey. And it surprised me when we realized our oldest daughter had some food allergies as well. We didn't realize it until she started to explain how much better her tummy felt. We immediately knew she was telling the truth when she had a "normal" meal outside of the house and was doubled over in stomach pain. Her reaction only pushed me harder to fight for health for all of us in the family, and I was pleased that they were all on board with me.

As much as I wanted my eye to heal quickly by adjusting my food, I knew there was more. I just didn't know what other options I had. One night, at our martial arts academy, I was explaining my situation to a fellow parent. Her recommendation was to take a holistic approach. She recommended a lady who studied and practiced a type of muscle testing. I had no idea what this was or how it worked, but I was open to all things at this point. Dr. Stewart had given me the go ahead to try anything and everything to heal this. Since there wasn't any current research studies being done, I had the green light to experiment on myself. So I did. I called immediately and was scheduled for a visit with this holistic practitioner. For the purpose of this book I am changing her actual name and will refer to her as Alice.

I was excited for my appointment. I had a great reference whom I trusted, and I had that bubbling vibration inside of me again, because I felt one step closer to my goal. I decided to go by myself to the first appointment. As much as my family was there to support me, I enjoyed doing some of these steps on my own to just clear my head. This was a good thing because my first appointment was a whirlwind.

I walked into the beautiful little building and was greeted by a staff wearing scrubs. My immediate reaction was an impressed shock. This place looked like a spa and everyone seemed so professional. It looked like everyone was a nurse or doctor of some kind. *This has to be my answer!* I thought without really understanding what they did or who they were. After filling out forms and doing some interesting spit tests and urine tests, I was finally able to see the holistic practitioner. At the time, though, since I knew nothing about this kind of work, I mistakenly thought she was a doctor of some sort. I later found out she wasn't, but my initial impression of a white coat threw me off.

Alice was absolutely beautiful. She was a petite, glowing angel in my eyes. Her skin was radiant and didn't have a flaw mark on it. She vibrated with energy and alertness, something I missed from my own life. I sat across the desk from her and explained my story. She wrote down all the details and gave me the hard facts. In a nutshell, most of her spit test results showed imbalances with my minerals in one way or another. She also labeled my gallbladder as a major organ that was affected, and she suggested that the scars I had on my body were blocking energy from traveling correctly.

None of this made sense to me, but I was willing to go along with it if that meant my eye would be healed. I lay on her massage-like table with my right arm raised right above my shoulder. She started pushing my arm down towards my hip really quickly with different bottles contain something inside of them. She explained that the technique she used helped her figure out what supplements my body needed. The technique of muscle testing was using the reflex in the muscle to either be strong or weak depending on how my system reacted to the small containers she had on me. She also said that I needed to do a liver/gallbladder cleanse; whatever that was. She made sure I had a clear schedule to do the cleanse because she said I would have to be in the bathroom the whole time clearing out "stones."

After I was done with the muscle testing portion, she rushed me out of the room as quickly as she could. She was on to the next patient and I was shuffled over to her staff. The two staff ladies had totally different personalities. One seemed sweet, but also unsure of herself. I picked up right away a sense of guilt, but I passed it off thinking it was sympathy for my situation. The other staff member

Clarity

was in charge of selling the supplements that Alice told me I needed. She was a stern lady who seemed to know her way around all of the supplements. She flew through the list Alice had given her, pulling bottle after bottle, and quickly rang me up. The total with all the supplements, visits, and other treatments came to over $1,000.00. They also wanted me to add on sessions with a healthcare counselor for an additional $240. This was really, really expensive! And why did I need a health counselor?! I was dumbfounded. Not to mention the bills were going to keep rolling in to keep up with these services. *How was I going to keep up with this expense?* I thought quietly. Something wasn't sitting right with me, but I reluctantly handed over my credit card and asked the lady to take off the counselor sessions.

  I was excited to start this journey. After all, I just spent a ton of money on this and I assumed this wasn't going to be that bad. Boy was I wrong. I started the supplement drops right away. They tasted horrible, but they surprisingly didn't seem to affect me too badly. I also started the process for the cleanse. I had no idea what I was getting myself into. The cleanse required me to drink Epsom salt multiple times throughout the day, without food, to clean out my intestines. After doing this for the day, I was instructed to drink olive oil and grapefruit juice to help push out the "stones." I'm going to save you from the gross details of this part, but all you need to know is, I thought I was going to die.

  My stomach had never been in so much pain. Half way through this "cleanse" I was standing in the kitchen, so weak I could barely hold myself up. Tears were running down my face and I realized this was a huge mistake. All of a sudden, I was getting flashbacks of high school and college when I struggled with eating. I had also developed IBS in college, which caused chronic constipation at times and then bouts of laxatives to help my system get back on track. This experience was like living that all over again.

  My husband came to my side and asked what was wrong. Crying uncontrollably, I said, "I am NEVER, NEVER, doing this again. I have worked so hard to learn about food the right way and how to get my stomach to process food correctly. I'm not afraid to eat any more and I will not let this trigger my eating disorder that I had in high school and college. I will not and cannot ever let my kids see me like this again! They don't need to think this is normal because it's not!" I collapsed in his arms, too weak to stand any more.

The next day, I made it out of the woods. The night had been painful and long, and, unfortunately, the bathroom was still my friend. I looked horrible, and I felt like I had the stomach flu. I gathered myself after a long day and headed to the school for work. Luckily, I didn't have to teach, but I knew I had done a number on my system when a male parent looked at me and with a surprised look said, "Are you feeling okay?! You don't look well." He was right, I didn't look well. I was defeated, weak, embarrassed, and ashamed.

I did some research on this cleanse and I got mixed reviews. Some said it was really important to do, others said it was dangerous. In the end, it didn't really matter what others wrote about. I was certain that this wasn't the option for me. My little voice inside of me was screaming! I wasn't going to ignore it this time! I finally knew I had to follow my heart and I would find the answers. I didn't know how exactly, but I knew I would figure it out.

My husband came to my next appointment with Alice. I brought all of my supplements with and all of my paperwork. We walked into the office and she was eager to put me on the table to get started right away. I stopped her and said, "Before we get started I have some questions for you." She looked at me with a flash of frustration. I continued, "I believe in what you're doing with the muscle testing, but I can't do another cleanse like this. I don't understand how this can be healthy for the intestines. Every time I would do this cleanse I will be flushing out all the bad bacteria as well as all the good bacteria. I know your recommendation is to keep doing these cleanses, but I won't do another one. The cleanse will trigger an unhealthy lifestyle that I've battled with at a younger time in my life. How can we move forward without doing that part?"

Her frustration turned to a slow burning anger. She became very firm with her delivery in saying, "Listen, Hunny, if you think this is going to be easy, you're sadly mistaken. I can't help you if you don't do these cleanses. This is why we recommended our health counselor. You obviously need to see her through this process.

Clarity

You're not going to get better unless you do these." I stared at her. Where was her compassion, kindness, and that glowing personality I had witnessed in my last visit? I stumbled on, "So you're saying this is the only way to work with you is if I do these cleanses? You don't believe that you can rebuild the intestinal wall with good bacteria? You only heal if you push out these 'stones'? Who's to say these 'stones' are actually what you say they are?"

She ended the intense conversation with telling me I was wasting her time. She showed us the door as she promised that I would have a refund waiting for me at the counter. That was a good thing because if she hadn't given me a refund, I would have told whomever was sitting in the waiting room to run. I reluctantly kept my mouth shut as I walked out. Emotions were raging inside of me. I was furious, confused, red-hot pissed off to say the least. The nice staff lady now showed her true colors, and I could tell her demeanor was truly guilt as she slinked around the waiting room trying not to make eye contact with me. How could they sell this program to people? Did they actually ever get better? The stern staff lady angrily took my card and my supplements and proceeded with my refund. We walked out of there feeling like we were just steamrolled.

I knew I was making the right decision for myself, but now I was filled with so many more questions. After researching gut health more on Dr. Axe's site, as well as others, I really felt like I had to rebuild my body, not put it through more stress with weird cleanses. That program would have become extremely stressful, and I needed the opposite of that. At this point, I kept on with eating as well as I could under the leaky gut protocol. I followed up for my next appointment with Dr. Stewart and found out that my eye had actually improved quite a bit. I still needed to have an injection, but the glimmer of hope helped me keep pushing forward. My stomach was feeling much better, and I was starting to get a nice glow back to my skin. Things were starting to look up until an annoying thought crossed my mind. Was my latest scan of my retina better because of the week I saw Alice, or was it better because of my eating. Time would tell.

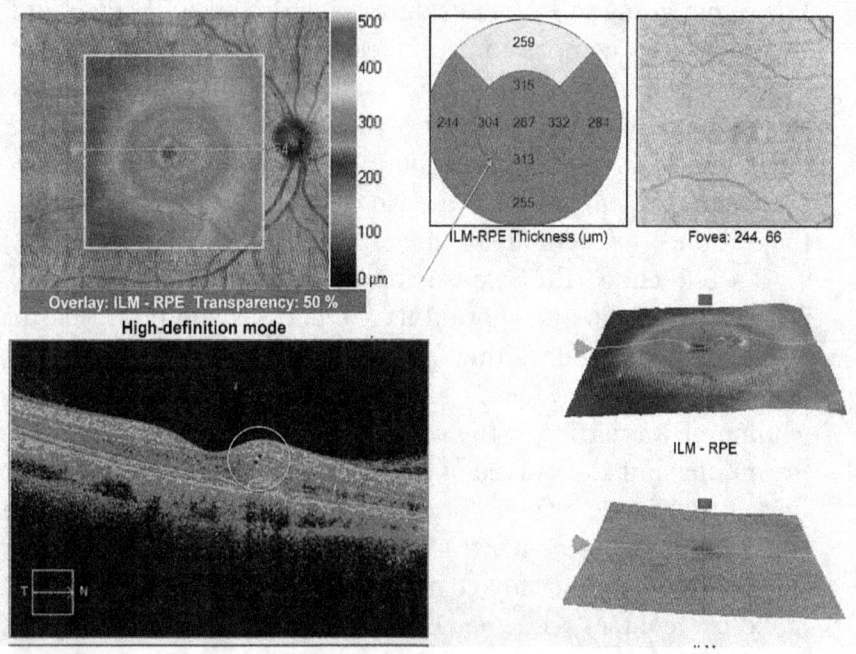

(Photo Caption: The OTC scan, 1/30/17, of the right eye showed a decrease in fluid pooling in the eye. The arrow shows the numbers decreased since the last scan.)

WHAT I DID AND WHAT YOU CAN DO: ACTION STEPS 9-12

> **Step 9 - Recognize Your Blessings:**

It's important to remember the happy things along the way. This sometimes can be really hard to do, especially if you're in the thick of putting all of the pieces together. Even though you'll feel this is difficult, talk to your cheerleader person about what's going right. If you can't find it in that moment, make sure to ask them to help you find it. When you can shift your mindset and stay in a positive motion-forward mentally, you're healing will speed up. We'll talk about this more in the next few chapters. For now, write down on a piece of paper what you're thankful for in the process that you're on right now. It can be really simple like, "I am thankful that I can still see." Or, it can be something really in depth like, "I am thankful that

I can see and continuing to find ways to help speed up the healing process." Another example would be, "I am grateful I'm still alive" instead of "I am grateful I'm not dead." Whatever you choose, just make sure it's written in a positive light. Speak from your heart and find joy in the accomplishments you've had this far.

> **Step 10 - Journal:**

This step is a great way for you to express what you're going through in the moment. Sometimes, getting your thoughts out on paper will help you connect the dots even further. It helps open up your mind in a way that helps you get off the mental hamster wheel and into a thought process of clear forwardness. The other aspect I'd like to encourage you to do, is to start a food journal. Often, when a person is having trouble with their health, they may notice issues with food as well. It's a great idea to document and start paying attention to your body on a deeper level. When you become in tune with what foods make you feel good after eating them and what foods make you feel bad after eating them, you'll start to awaken a part of you that you didn't know existed. This step is all about helping you focus on your inner body more and diving deeper within for the answers. Starting with food is a great place to evaluate what you're putting in your body. How your body handles food is a great clue to how your body is processing its nutrients.

> **Step 11 - Eat Organic:**

There's a saying that goes, "What you put in is what you get out." This is so true to the body. If you're putting in pizza and drinking pop every night, you're not going to get out a high functioning body that can walk up a flight of stairs and feel great. Nope! Pizza and Pop equal Poop. Yup, poop. You'll literally feel like poop if you keep eating that way. Now imagine you have a diet that's free from chemicals. Your food is exactly how it was intended to be. Free from pesticides, fertilizers, and GMOs. Our food these days has been so altered that it doesn't even classify as food any more. My suggestion is to slowly start to transition to organic and start to take notice of how your body feels.

For example, my husband didn't believe this type of eating would really do anything. He thought it was "hogwash" as he called it. So I asked him to eat organic with me as much as he could. I would cook all the meals and see what he thought after a few weeks. Amazingly, he said the food tasted so much more vibrant. The ultimate realization for him was when he ate a few "regular" strawberries, the kind that had chemicals and whatever else was concocted on there. Within minutes, his tongue was burning and he couldn't eat any more. He only had two or three medium-sized strawberries. He tried drinking some water, but the burning sensation lasted for a few hours. The next night, he ate some organic strawberries and the reaction didn't happen. It was an eye-opener for sure, but some people just need to witness things for themselves to believe it, which is perfectly fine. I'm proud of him for trying and recognizing the difference. He was now tapping into his body and listening to it.

Along with switching to organic, I also started juicing my veggies and fruits. This was a great way for my body to quickly absorb the nutrients from the food. If you like to juice, I would recommend investing in a good juicer. You'll get a lot more juice out of it than you would if you bought a cheaper one. I found that juicing really helped my intestines heal, and it also gave my skin a nice glow. You could also look at buying a green powder supplement that has loads of veggies in it as well. Make sure to do your homework with each supplement and to buy organic. For more ideas and information, you can visit my website at nikkiengels.com/products.

> **Step 12 - Follow Your Heart:**

Throughout my story, you've probably noticed my struggle in listening to my inner voice. That piece of you that you can hear, that constantly talks to you like a record player, that's your heart talking. Sometimes, your brain can override your thoughts and push down what your heart is really trying to say. This happened a few times in my story, when I felt one way but I ignored it and did the opposite. Most of the time, I regretted that decision. Within the last section, I finally listened to my voice and stood up for what I felt was right for me. Even though this holistic program I tried might have

Clarity

helped other people, I couldn't let that sway me from what was right for me. My heart screamed to try another way, and I'm so thankful I did. It led me on the path that I was supposed to be on, and that experience taught me an invaluable lesson to keep listening inward.

In this step, I want to encourage you to start listening in. Whatever decision you have in front of you, focus on your voice and follow it. If you're struggling with this, place your hands on your heart, close your eyes, and ask your question. Your answer will come to you faster than you can get the question out. That's your heart talking and you need to follow it. This is your body's way of helping you heal and navigate through all the decisions. Your heart will pick the right one, if you allow it to.

This step will take some practice to really hear yourself and what you need. Learn from your mistakes, recognize when you should have listened to the voice and didn't, and take action in knowing that the answers are within you, as you move forward with your decisions. It's up to you to heal your body, and it takes a lot of love and belief to get there. Remember, your heart knows the way and keep the saying in your mind when you have to make a decision, "Follow your heart." Do this and you'll stay on the best path for you.

** YOUR TO-DO LIST **

9. WRITE DOWN YOUR BLESSINGS, BIG AND SMALL.
10. START A JOURNEY JOURNAL AND/OR FOOD JOURNAL.
11. START SWITCHING YOUR FOOD AND BODY PRODUCTS TO ORGANIC.
12. FOCUS INWARDLY DAILY TO HEAR YOUR HEART SPEAK YOUR TRUTH.

Chapter 5: Cutting the Stress

I was feeling really good about my progress. Things seemed to be looking up, since my last scan looked quite a bit better. I still had a lot of inflammation in the eye, but, overall, the fluid hole wasn't presenting itself that much. I continued with my super clean eating and sticking to the foods that I knew I could have. This had its challenges at times, but, overall, it was worth it. I had to make a few adjustments when going to family gatherings or restaurants. I would either bring my own food, or, at a restaurant, I would try and order something that still somewhat aligned with what I was already doing. This got very challenging and was extremely stressful for my family. I was so dedicated to making my eye heal, however, that I kept a positive attitude as much as I could about the adversity. I also kept up on juicing every day and drinking detox teas. I kept searching for other answers in the process. My body was definitely responding positively to the changes I made. I now was getting compliments on my glowing skin, my energy was starting to come back, and I felt my sadness starting to leave me.

In the meantime, I had my home water tested to see if there were any toxic chemicals in it from the house fire, and I started to play with sitting in saunas after increasing my fluid intake. I was willing to try anything and everything to detox all the crap out of my system. All of these measures didn't result in any clues to the root cause of my eye misbehaving, unfortunately. My water tests came back fine and the saunas only seemed to make me sick afterwards. I knew my not feeling well could be part of the detox process, but it wasn't sitting well in my heart. I decided to table those ideas, as life got really crazy again and eating well seemed to be the best thing at the time.

    We decided to discontinue teaching students at the martial arts school who wanted to be professional fighters. Our satellite martial arts school in a different town also came to an end around this time. I also said goodbye to a loving career of portrait and wedding photography. Each of these aspects were hard to say goodbye to, and, although we were sad to see them go, we knew it was the right decision. The stress of all of them got to be too much, and we needed to refocus on what was important to our family. Even though we shifted this portion of our life, it didn't change the fact that things were still extremely stressful for us, and I felt like I was drowning in worry and anxiety from not having these three hubs of income anymore.

    Living in a small tourist town definitely has its challenges. Although we always seemed to maintain our expenses well in the past, our little coffee shop wasn't keeping up currently. The summers were great when our quaint town was filled with tourists and income was flowing in, but the long winters were money sucks. Our customers were wonderful and they really valued the coffee, but there just wasn't enough traffic to keep up with all the overhead expenses. Every month the bills would come in and the revenue was just not there to pay them. With our savings being depleted, we knew we had to make a change again. Our first thought was to invest more money into the business and build a new building, but that idea was more expensive than we could afford at the time. We also thought about closing for the winter, but we felt a responsibility to stay open for our staff. No matter which way we looked at it, we lost in one way or another. The stress I took on was a heavy load of optionless ideas. We were stuck with the property and business, and since we didn't have a winning solution at the time, we decided to get through another summer and hopefully recoup some of our winter expenses. (After that summer, we decided to shut down the coffee shop since the stress wasn't helping me in any way. We ate the costs and moved on.)

    It was now March of 2017, nine months from my impossible diagnosis. Our kids were now seven, five, and three and were all adjusting well to the weird adapted life shifts that had happened within the last few months. In these nine months, I had really taken on the approach that happiness needed to be the forefront of my mind. If something made me feel gross inside, I would say no. If something made me excited and alive, I would say yes. This happiness search not only applied to cutting out parts of business that caused stress, but it also went as far as saying yes or no to places I would get invited to, or to people who wanted to talk to me. I was constantly using my own heart calibration to lead me to where I needed to go. My mission was to stay in a stress-free zone, or as close to it as possible. If I didn't stay in a stress-free zone, my body would react immediately with nerve pain and an intense pressure behind the right eye.

My husband and I had our 10-year anniversary coming up in May that year. We had gotten married in Hawaii back in 2007 and it had been a long time since we had been back to the island. We had kicked the idea around about going back for our anniversary, but with where we were financially with the coffee shop, I didn't see how that was going to happen.

Despite my negative feelings about the coffee shop, I had this huge desire to plant my feet back in the magical land of Hawaii. My past trips to this remarkable place always made me feel like I was home. I'm not Hawaiian and I've never lived there, but I've traveled there multiple times in my life. Each time I went to Hawaii, I felt an immediate connection with the land. With each visit, I felt a part of me stayed there. I always felt this magnetic pull to the island and I always felt alive and free when I was surrounded by its lush green mountains, sparkling blue oceans, and its brave midnight black lava rock.

I sat on my couch one evening while Gary was still at the academy. I had just done another search for things to help my eye and felt content with the research that I had just found. It was a moment of quiet, since the kids had fallen asleep on the way home from running errands. The idea of Hawaii tantalized my imagination again. I closed my eyes and felt the strong longing feeling of going back. In my mind, I could hear the music, smell the flowers, and see all the smiles from the beautiful Hawaiian people.

Clarity

The thoughts and images came to my mind like a waterfall filling a lake. They poured in as I could feel the sand and hear the ocean waves. I slowly opened my eyes only to be transported back to my living room. Outside was snow covered, and I was feeling the effects of the frigid air as I sat in my house with piles of clothes layered on me.

My fingers suddenly reacted to the visions and started typing in information about flights. I couldn't handle the thought of not seeing this beautiful place again. I stopped for a brief moment and the thought came over me, "What if I lose my sight? I would regret not seeing all of that amazing beauty one last time." Tears started to roll down my face as I felt the pulling sensation to continue my online search for flights.

Flights were not cheap and I knew I wanted my whole family to go. I wanted those memories with my children just in case the worst happened. After searching and seeing the prices of tickets, I realized this was almost impossible. Our spring break week was only three weeks out and I had to plan according to our martial arts school's calendar and for our children's school schedules as well. Even though I felt a little defeated, a little voice inside toyed with me. In a sweet whisper I heard, "Just keep looking, get creative, you'll find a way."

Now that I had learned a little more to follow my heart, I put my fingers back on the keyboard. "Yes! I can figure this out. I don't know how, but I will!" Happiness was in the driver's seat like a kid on Christmas morning. Suddenly, I remembered that I hadn't looked at my frequent flyer mile points in quite some time. I raced over to the site and saw the amount. My mouth literally fell open! I had 500,000 points! We hadn't used the points in years, and I had no idea we had accumulated so many. It was like a gift from the universe! I couldn't believe when I plugged in the dates and my balance due was zero! I even had enough points to bring along my mother-in-law, Teresa, to help with the kids, since they were so little.

I felt the excitement and bubbling joy building inside me like a geyser that was happy and alive. "Oh my gosh, oh my gosh!" I yelled out, forgetting the kids were asleep. I called my husband and said as calmly as possible, "Hi, Hunny! What do you think about going to Hawaii in three weeks?" He answered back as fast as humanly possible, "What?! Really?! Ummm yeah!!" Then he started to ask the obvious question, "How can we afford it? Is that too soon? Are you sure you want to do this? Can we leave the businesses?" I really hadn't thought much farther than just going, but I figured we could figure out the rest. I hung up the phone while leaving the idea hanging out there.

The next day, I called my mother-in-law. She answered the phone and I blurted out to her, "Hey, want to come to Hawaii with the family?!" She's a "yes woman" so she immediately agreed right away. Then she chuckled and said, "Let me check with my husband quick, I'm hopping on a plane in Florida to come home as we speak." I knew her chuckle was from excitement, and she couldn't pass up an opportunity like this. She, of course, said yes once she got home.

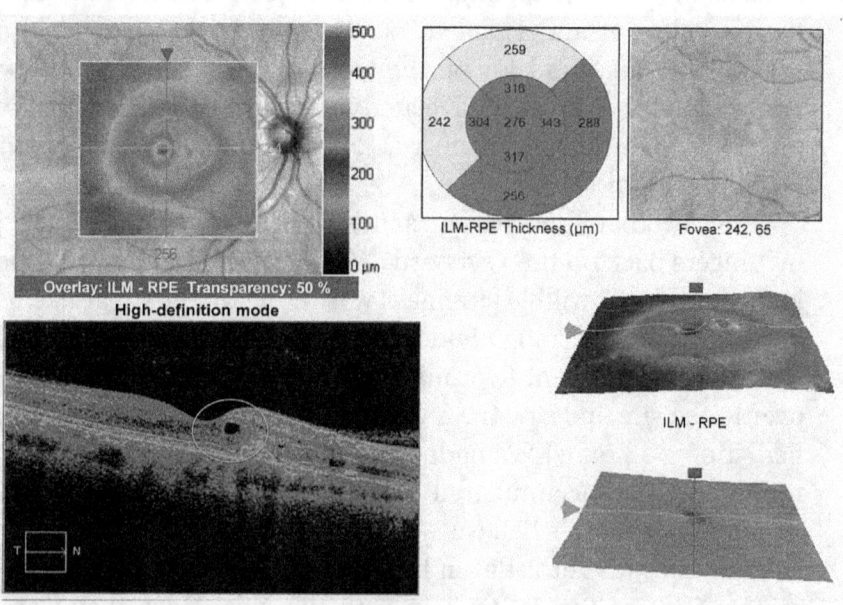

Photo Caption: The OTC scan, taken on 3/13/17 shows the condition of the eye had gotten a little worse.)

Clarity

Everything seemed to align perfectly. I had an appointment with Dr. Stewart in the middle of March, and we were leaving a week later. At the appointment, I made sure to explain to him that we were leaving and to get the okay to fly and travel with the condition my eye was in. I was hoping I got the okay, since I had already booked the tickets and planned everything! I was a little disappointed that the scan came back worse than the previous scan, but the doctor wasn't alarmed and said I was doing fine with pushing my injections to six weeks in between.

He also explained that there were lots of retinal specialists I could see on Oahu, HI if something happened during our time there. I also started to explain to him some of the symptoms I was having from the injections. I further explained how I was feeling a little better after I changed my diet. He politely said, "I don't think it's going to do much for your condition, but keep on doing it. It can't hurt anything." I also told him why I wanted to go to Hawaii, and he said, "Yes, keep living your life. Don't let this disease control what you want to do." And just like that, he smiled, shook our hands, and said, "Safe travels and have a great time." I still had to get an injection, but this one didn't bother me as much. I was going to Hawaii in a week and as I got the injection, I kept thinking of the beautiful place that awaited me.

We arrived in Hawaii after a long traveling day. Even though our flights were paid for with frequent flyer miles, we weren't awarded the best flights or anything. In fact, traveling this way, we had to be okay with getting weird flight times and multiple layovers. Honestly, I didn't care. I was going to my favorite place to be enriched by its healing powers. It's funny to write that now because I didn't know much about the healing powers at the time, but I knew they were there instinctively. Before we arrived, I had this feeling like I was meant to go. Everything lined up so perfectly that I had to follow this instinctive thought. I looked up a few places that I wanted to go and I made a check list of all the places to visit that would heal me. My main purpose was to have fun, let my hair down, and just breathe in all the beauty around me.

Since we arrived early in the evening, Hawaii time, we were absolutely exhausted from our 24 hours of straight travel time.

Everyone seemed to bounce back pretty fast from the jet lag, except for myself. Once we landed I started to see black floaters flying everywhere in my right eye. Floaters were pretty common for me these days. It was scary when they first happened since they often looked like a floating, black bug, the size of a blackfly. Unfortunately, this was a common side effect from the medication and it was something that would come and go. These floaters were quite different, though, and it scared me. My eye felt a little different inside after landing and the images were like little black sparkles, danced around my eyeball. They were making me really dizzy. I even tried to stand up out of my seat on the plane, only to realize I was forced back down from the spins. I started to worry that the pressure change from flying hurt my inner eye somehow. This wasn't how I wanted to start out this trip. I wasn't going to let this stop me! My anxiety flared up as I tried to push forward while gathering my belongings and exited the plane.

Gary and Teresa kept asking me if I were alright. I must have been wearing the expression of panic on my face. Slowly the floaters disappeared and I could breathe a little. I knew I needed to get some sleep, but I couldn't wait to see the ocean. We stayed in a cute little house in Kailua, where the beach was within walking distance. We literally dropped our bags off, put on our suits, and headed for the silky sand and crazy blue waves. Walking to the beach I was taken aback. As the trees separated, the beauty of the brilliant blue water was more magnificent than I had remembered. I took it all in as I stood there: the smell of saltwater in the air, the mist of the ocean bathing my face, and the warm sand traveling up my body like a cozy blanket!

I sat with Gary for a moment as Teresa played with the kids in the ocean. It was so nice to have a minute to talk to him. He asked how I was doing. I didn't lie; I explained that I felt like a train ran over me. He looked at me and said, "Switch it. Try and shake it off; you can do it. Maybe playing with the kids will help." I looked at him like he was crazy, but I knew deep down he was right. "Okay," I answered back. I pulled myself up even though my whole body wanted to just lay there and melt into a puddle of exhaustion. I started to walk toward the ocean where the kids happily greeted me.

Clarity

Their little faces and big, bright smiles brought energy to my body. They grabbed hands, along with mine, and instructed me to jump over the waves as they crashed on the beach. Each jump I made, my body felt like I was stuck to the ground. It felt as if I had pounds and pounds of lead chains on my feet. Then something magical started to happen. With every jump, with every moment the water hit my feet, and with the kid's happiness surrounding me, I started to feel slightly better. It was like pure magic. Jump, shed negative energy, jump, and shed more! The next thing I knew, the kids and I were running up and down the beach trying to play tag with the waves. In that moment, I knew this trip was going to make me stronger, wiser, and healthier.

We had two weeks to explore the island, but I knew this time would go quickly. I started my plan with taking the family to all the places I had noted before we arrived. I wanted our kids to understand the culture and the beauty within and why I was so drawn to it. Everything we did they found happiness in, and so did I. With each day that passed, I felt that little kid in me starting to shine from the inside out. We all did, honestly.

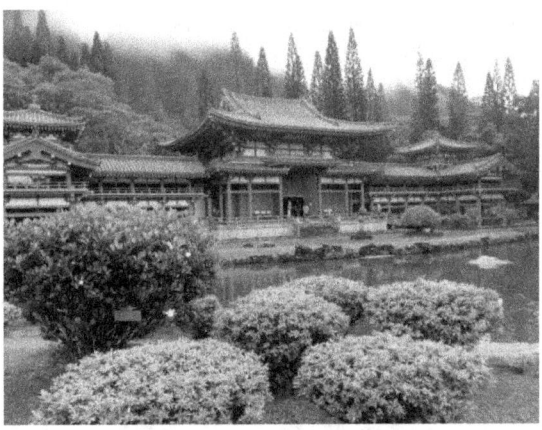

(Photo Caption: The Byodo-In Temple in Oahu, HI)

One of our stops on the list was the Byodo-In Temple. I wasn't quite sure what to expect with this stop, but it blew my expectations out of the water. Here sat a beautiful temple underneath the Ko'olau Mountains. According to their website "The Byodo-In Temple is a non-practicing Buddhist temple which welcomes people of all faiths to worship, meditate, or to simply appreciate its beauty."[11] But for me, this temple was a place of peace and healing. I felt a buzz of positive energy as I walked through the grounds. I took it all in again as I looked up at the large, red temple beneath the contrasting lush green mountains.

We made our way to a large bell that sat on the left side of the temple. According to the temple's website, "The bell is customarily rung before one enters the temple to spread the eternal teachings of Buddha. Ringing the bell will purify the mind of evil spirits and temptation. It is said that ringing this bell will bring you happiness, blessings, and a long life. It is customarily rung before entering the temple."[12] As I rang the bell, I felt a warm relaxation come over me.

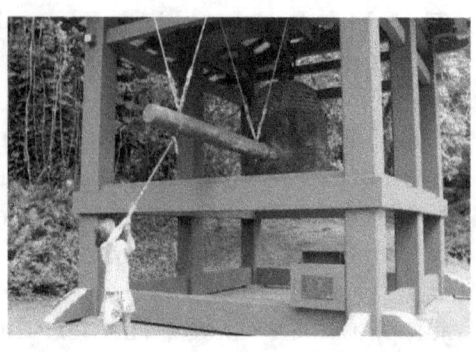

(Photo Caption: Sada, Nikki's oldest daughter, rings the bell that invites blessings.)

That was what I needed on this trip. I welcomed anything that helped my healing, and good blessings were exactly what I was looking for. After ringing the bell, we proceeded to the temple where a large Buddha sat in the middle of the room. Walking in, my nose was hit with the smell of incense burning and the smell of musty old books, yet no books were seen in this vast space.

The Buddha was breathtaking with its large golden body sitting on top of a lotus flower. There was a spiritual and honorable feeling that lurked in the room. I watched as visitor after visitor walked up to the towering Buddha, lit an incense, and silently said a prayer.

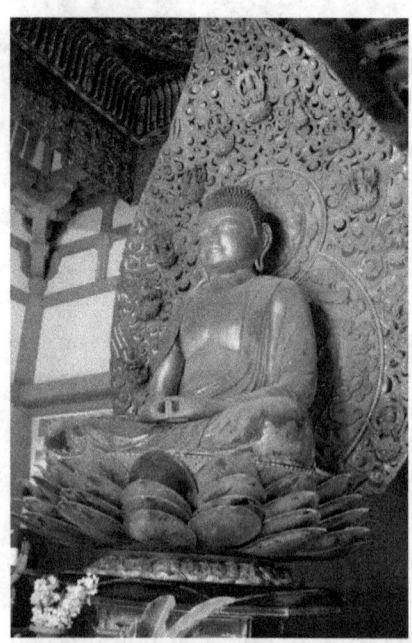

(Photo Caption: Photo taken by Nikki Engels of the Buddha figure within the Byodo-In Temple. The Buddha was carved by Masuzo Inui.)

Clarity

The cold concrete floor nudged my feet to move forward. I felt the urge to take part, but I was also feeling extremely vulnerable. I knew nothing about this temple, and I knew nothing about the Buddha. Yet, I felt the urge to say my wishes to him as if he were begging me to speak. I walked up to a beautifully set table in front of the Buddha, lit an incense, and clearly spoke the words in my head, "Please allow me to find a way to heal my eye, and find clarity in the situation that I am in." I put the incense in the dish to burn and slowly stepped away. I suddenly felt like crying.

Emotions were running over me like a stone stuck in a stream. I held it together, but I knew this moment was a powerful one. I didn't know if the way I prayed was correct, but I felt an inspired hope covering me. It felt as if the hope was lightly sprayed on my body for only me to feel. It was a magical day to say the least and the magic kept on spreading.

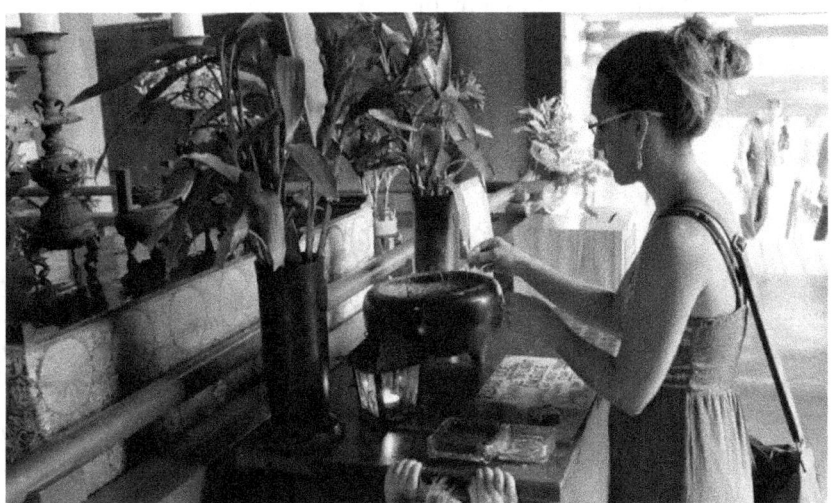

(Photo Captured: Nikki sets a lighted incense into the bowl as she says a prayer. Her prayer was "Please allow me to find a way to heal my eye, and find clarity in the situation that I am in.)

WHAT I DID AND WHAT YOU CAN DO: ACTION STEPS 13-16

> **Step 13 - Cut the Stress:**

In this step, I encourage you to ask yourself the hard questions about your life. We all have stress in different ways, but you'll have to determine which stresses you would love to get rid of. Take a bird's eye view of your life and make another web. This web will be called your Stress Web. For a free downloadable Stress Web, visit my website at www.nikkiengels.com/downloads. In the middle of your web is the word stress. On the outside of your web list all of the things in your life that cause you stress. The only rule for this is to think big. For example, I could write all the little things that bothered me about the coffee shop; like making sure it was cleaned, making sure it was staffed, did the staff show up on time, did they need change, etc. But for this challenge, I want you to think bigger. On my web, I listed the Coffee Shop, Pro Fighters, Photography, Money, Certain People/Relationships, etc. Now under each one of these big items list how your life would change if you didn't have this stress in your life any more. Once you have that, list three steps on how you can cut it out of your life.

This part isn't going to be easy and you'll want to have your life partner to help you with these decisions. A big part of your healing is to welcome a new way of thinking, and that's going to require you to make some physical changes in the process. With your life partner or your elected cheerleader, talk about each one and discuss how things could be better without some of these constant stresses. Once you make a plan, put it into place by trying to cut out at least two of your stressors. Your body will thank you for it, and, mentally, you'll start to feel lighter. Taking decisive action in your healing, helps anchor your commitment and belief in yourself. There is a great quote by Albert Einstein that says, "Insanity is doing the same thing over and over again, but expecting different results." So rip off the band aid and start making the hard changes you need to in order to speed up your healing.

➢ **Step 14 - Do the Hard Work:**
You'll need to make some big changes to the negative aspects of your life, but that doesn't mean you get to slack off with the things you already set in motion. Nope! In order to heal your condition, stay positive and understand that you'll need to stay consistent in being dedicated to fixing your problem. At times, you're going to be tired and feel like this is so much work, or maybe other family and friends won't understand why you're drastically changing your food habits and you're sick of hearing their questions. Remember this, as my husband always says, "You don't want it to be easy; you want it to be worth it." Remember, a day will come when you'll look back and thank yourself for doing all the hard work.

In this step, write down all the little milestones that you've hit so far and celebrate your little wins. Even if this is just listing why you're stressed or maybe you've recognized an event that triggered a negative emotion within. This may seem small, but really you're on a path to a greater success. You have to allow yourself to be content with all the little successes along the way. These little successes will lead to your big success of healing.

➢ **Step 15 - Do What Makes You Happy:**
Find your happy! This doesn't mean forcing a smile on your face, or lie and tell everyone you're fine when really, you're crushed inside. This really means to sit down and ask yourself what you want to do, see, or experience. We as humans are meant to grow and expand. It's what the universe wants us to do. If we just stayed in the same job, the same place in life, and never pushed forward with new experiences, a piece of us dies.

For me, this meant that I had to travel to Hawaii. There, my expanded knowledge led me to my next pathway. You don't have to travel, though. Maybe, for you, it's something simpler. It could be trying a new food, going zip lining, skydiving, hiking a new path in the woods, taking a weekend trip to a little town you've never been to before. It doesn't matter what it is. The only rule is to do something that makes you feel excited again! It has to be something that gets the thrilling emotions from the inside out. Your goal is to feel like a kid again and rediscover the part of you that has been missing for so long. You might be surprised what you discover about yourself and clues to help you heal in unexpected places.

➢ **Step 16 - Be Open to New Thinking:**
When you're expanding your newfound you with your happy quest, be open to all of the new ways of thinking around you. When I walked into the temple, I had no idea what it symbolized, or how it could help. I had no idea if I was even praying right or who I was praying to in that moment. I just knew there was magic there. I could feel it. I stayed open to all ways of thinking, because, surely, I didn't have the answers at the time to fully heal my eye. I gave my trust into the greater good of the universe to help me on the path. In the process, I found a connection to other people who had experiences or wisdom that helped me along the way.

This is a great time to be inspired. If you come to a new way of thinking that doesn't align with your values, take the time to ask yourself why they don't. Also ask, is there anything in this that I do find value in. Even if it's something small like ringing a large bell. When you're open to new ideas, your body and mind become open to new ways of healing as well. Again, I think of the Einstein quote I wrote about earlier. Sometimes, it takes a different approach to find your needed answers.

** YOUR TO-DO LIST **

13. MAKE YOUR STRESS WEB AND START CROSSING OFF THE STRESSORS.
14. CELEBRATE YOUR WINS AS YOU CONTINUE YOUR HARD WORK.
15. LISTEN TO THE KID IN YOU AND LET THAT PERSON DRIVE.
16. STAY FLUID IN YOUR THOUGHTS AND EXPERIENCES, LEARN FROM ALL THINGS.

Chapter 6: Finding Outside Help

      The next few days only got better. The more time we spent on the island, the more I felt free and alive. I could feel the stress just slipping away from me. We decided to do a few activities where we would need to be in or around water. I was nervous about this part of the trip because I still wasn't able to wear my contacts. My eye doctors and my sister Malina, who worked in optical, had diligently worked with me to get my eyes to see a balanced image. Before the trip, we finally figured out that I needed a prism in my glasses. This adjustment helped the muscles in my eyes work together again. We assumed that the scar tissue in the right eye, from the rupturing blood vessel, had now formed a new problem with my sight. This was a little easier to correct than the bleed, but it also meant that wearing contacts wouldn't be possible. Unfortunately, contacts couldn't be made with a prism correction so my only option was glasses, or wear contacts that made me feel like I was looking through a fishbowl.

      I had packed a few pairs of contacts for the trip, since I knew we would be doing some activities, like petting a dolphin at the marina and snorkeling, where I wouldn't be allowed to wear glasses. I put my contacts in that morning before we left for the marina. It had been nine months since wearing them. It felt odd and strange to have them in my eyes, but I also felt a sense of freedom by not having my glasses on my face. My eyes were struggling to put together an image that wasn't distorted. I felt like vomiting the whole way to the marina, but slowly things started to get better. By the time we got there, I was doing pretty good. I could notice some distortion but only if I focused on it.

I ended up wearing my contacts the rest of the day, even though I didn't have to. I was amazed that I could see so well. I had tried wearing my contacts back home a few times, but I had to take them out immediately because of how bad the images were. This was a completely different experience. The next day, we decided to go snorkeling and I put my contacts in again. This time, my eyes worked even better in them than the day before. It was surprising and exciting! I had no idea what was happening, but my spirits were soaring from the hope and these moments of success.

We also traveled to a place called Waimea Valley where our family could hike back to a waterfall. I remembered doing this hike in the past and some of the visitors were swimming in the pool underneath the falls. I always wanted to do this, but I never did. This time, it was on my list of adventures. Plus, I wanted the kids to experience it as well. We all were a little on the crabby side that day. I know it seems impossible to be crabby in Hawaii, but for some reason, our moods were a little off. We decided to try and shake it off by doing this gentle hike. This place was a magical botanical garden. Everywhere we turned we were looking at bright, brilliant flowers and lush green leaves. There were plants from all corners of the world. And this place was filled with Hawaiian history. We could feel the presence of ancient wisdom among us.

Once we reach the waterfall, we were pleasantly surprised that they had a lifeguard station there with life vests. This was great for us since I wanted the kids to experience swimming in a waterfall. My mother-in-law decided to stay out of the water with our son, who was too scared and little to try the experience. My husband and I entered the ice cold freshwater pool. It was freezing, but soon our bodies adjusted to the sensation. I was very cautious the whole time in the pool as to not splash any water on my face. Since I was getting injections, I had to be extremely careful not to put anything in my eye because of the possible risk for infection. Since we were all floating in peace we all looked up. The cliffs above us were looking down on us like gods. I felt the presence of a magical energy again. The longer I looked around, the more I realized how thankful I was for this moment. I tried to etch the images of the cliffs and waterfall in my mind so that I would remember it forever. I didn't want to

Clarity

ever lose this moment. I was in such a historical place with my family, swimming in a bath of natural energy, being kissed by my favorite star, while green jungle surrounded us. This was remarkable and it made the kid in me squeal in delight.

We exited the falls, returned our life vests, and started our walk back to the front of the park. Gary, the girls, and I were all giggly and happy. It was as if someone had flipped a switch and recharged our batteries. I also noticed that my son and mother-in-law were still in a similar mood as when we had gotten there. It wasn't bad, but it wasn't energetic and full of energy like our transformed personalities were. This was very interesting to me and I made a mental note of it. Interestingly enough, this same phenomenon happened again on another day.

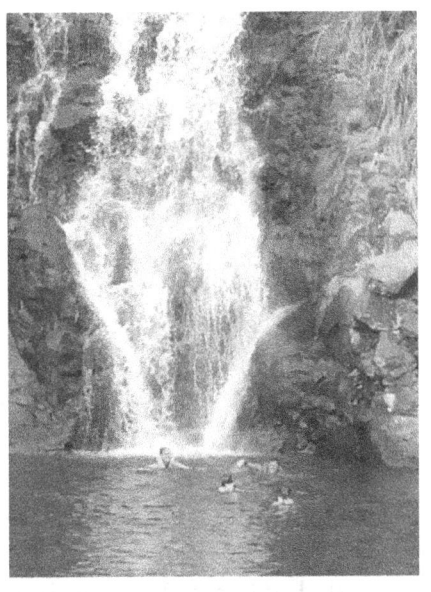

(Photo Caption: Nikki, Gary, and their two daughters, Sada and Ree swim in the Waimea Falls. Photo taken by Teresa Lorenz.)

This time it was with the ocean water. Something was starting to click for me. I could wear my contacts here, I felt like the water held magic energy, and we were all looking and feeling younger. I couldn't see the magic, but I could feel it everywhere.

We had about a week and a half left on the trip and I wore my contacts almost the entire time. I also realized that my nerve pain was gone and my back/side pain also had vanished. I mentioned

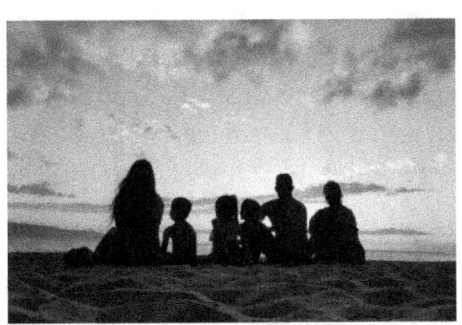

(Photo Caption: Nikki and her family, Dez, Ree, Sada, Gary, and Teresa sit on the beach looking out at the beautiful sunset over the ocean.)

something to my husband about it and he agreed. He felt healthier and younger as well, but he was amazed at how well my eye was doing. That was more of a surprise to him than anything else. He also mentioned that I was like a different person there. I was free, light, and overall happier.

Two days before we had to leave this beautiful place, my emotions started to grip on my heart. I didn't want to leave. I didn't want to face the stressful life that was waiting for me back home. I dreaded every thought of it, and it saddened me to only have two more days in this magical place. The longing feeling started to creep in every time we would drive by the ocean. I had a great life back home, don't get me wrong, but it wasn't relaxing by any means. I had so many thoughts swirling around my head. What projects did we have to get done before summer and after summer, what else did I have to do to heal my eye, and what are we going to do with the dreaded coffee shop? The list went on and on in my head. I was guilty of letting my thoughts steer my emotions over a cliff.

The night before we left for home, my eye started to ache. I felt like I had gotten punched in the eye. I also noticed my vision had started to shift again. I felt the worry and panic hit my gut like a rock or hard brick. My body also started to ache again. I didn't want to face the music when I got home, but I knew in my heart that my eye was in trouble again. It had only been four weeks since my last injection, but I could tell I needed to be seen right away.

Once we were home, I called Dr. Stewart and hesitantly told his receptionist that I needed to be seen right away. They got me in the next day and, sure enough, my retina had created a hole as if I had waited a full six weeks. The doctor was a little taken aback by it, but the same treatment was required and he said we would see what would happen the next month. He didn't think it was from traveling in a plane. In fact, he basically stated that he didn't have a good explanation for why blood vessels do this, they just do sometimes. He didn't have an explanation for why I could wear my contacts in Hawaii either.

His nonexplanation really got under my skin. How could there not be a good reason for this? My scans were getting better and now they were going completely the other way. I was so defeated and frustrated again. I had just left a place where I could see perfectly fine for about a week and a half; I came home, and now not only can I not wear my contacts again, but my retina had misbehaved again! I was beyond confused and so was my husband. We again were left with unanswered questions and puzzling thoughts.

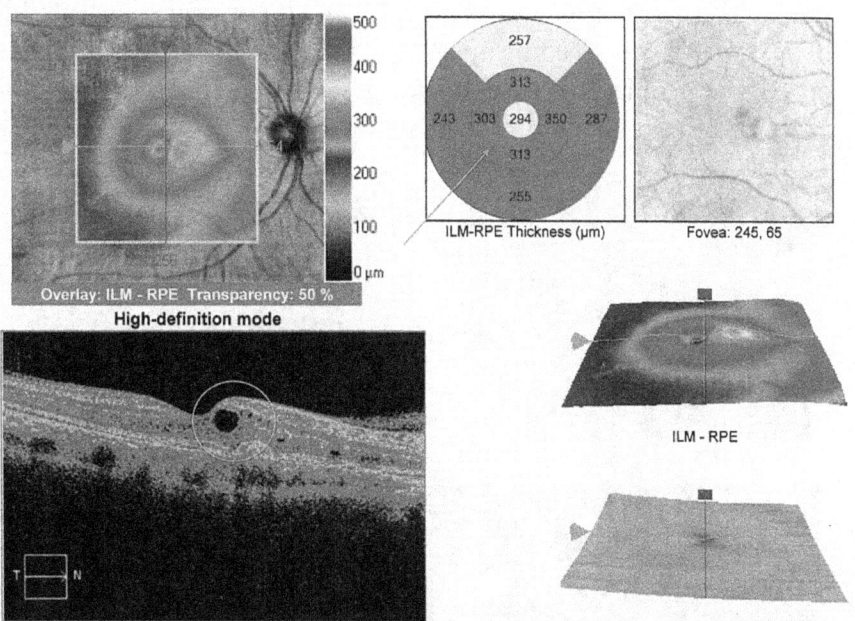

(Photo Caption: OTC Scan taken 4/10/17. The fluid has expanded and the numbers are reflecting the negative change.)

As we drove home from the injection appointment, I asked Gary in an irate tone if I were going crazy. I said, "I don't get it! How could I see in Hawaii, but not here? Am I missing something? Like really, be honest with me!"

He looked over at me with loving eyes and said in a calm voice, "You're not crazy. Something happened there. We all saw it. You were a different person there and your eye was definitely better. I can't put my finger on it, but something in Hawaii allowed you to see differently." His words hit my heart like pulsing hugs. That was exactly what I wanted to hear. I wasn't crazy, but I was more confused.

Four weeks and two days had passed and I again had to hightail it into Dr. Stewart's office. My scans were even worse. I was losing ground and fast. I started looking through all of my scans. I became a detective with each number, and asked Dr. Stewart all the questions I could think of regarding the images. I analyzed and tracked where the fluid was coming in, and how it was accumulating in the eye. All I could come up with was that it was getting worse and now I was facing Dr. Stewart's suggestion of getting an injection every two weeks! I couldn't let that happen.

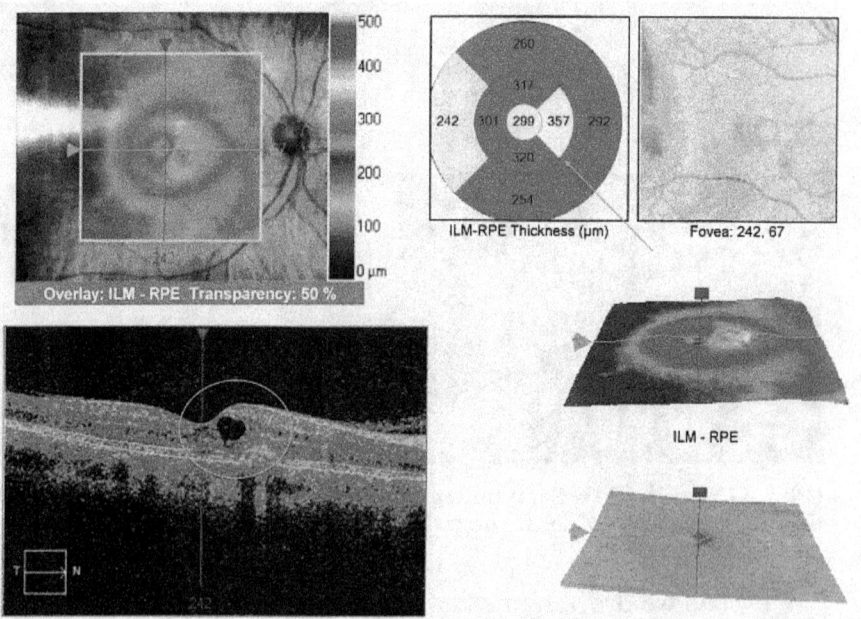

(Photo Caption: OCT Scan from 5/10/17 shows the fluid is continually getting worse.)

My thoughts and research started to question what I had done with Alice again. Yup, that pesky thought of whether she had really helped with her wild protocol entered my mind. This thought infuriated me because there was no way I was going back there, nor would she take me back. But the thought kept lurking in my mind and the research kept coming up without answers. I happened to be talking to a friend during one of my daughters' dance practices. I was telling her my short version of the story and she immediately

Clarity

asked if I was talking about Alice. Surprised and a little embarrassed, I said yes. She told me that she had been going to her as well. Her experience had been the same, but most of the appointments were for her daughter. It turned out that she also knew a different lady by the name of Jennifer (name was changed for this book) who practiced muscle testing about an hour from our town. She supposedly did the same approach Alice swore by, but was a lot more compassionate towards her clients. She also said she didn't make her clients do the liver/gallbladder cleanse. After hearing this information, it sounded like exactly what I wanted.

    I went home that night and explained to Gary that I was going to do this. His puzzled look made me explain further. "I have to do something, Hunny! I've literally looked at these scans over and over again. Something happened with the Alice appointment, but I don't fully understand what. I'm going to set this up and just see what she says." He was supportive, but I could tell he was a bit concerned.

    I went into see Jennifer on May 11th, 2017. She worked in a cute and professional private office. As I walked into the waiting room, I could tell this was going to be a totally different experience. The place was decorated with class and it smelled of sweet essential oils, neither one were over the top. The staff was great and very welcoming as I sat down to wait. Jennifer came out right away. I could tell she had a sweet and compassionate personality. Even though this was my first impression, I made sure to not be fooled like I had been with Alice. At least this time around, I knew a little more than before. Since time for my eye was of the essence, I didn't want to be fooled again, so I left out the information about my Alice experience. I felt shady doing this, but I really wanted her honest explanation of what she did before I decided to work with her. I felt like this information would only muck up the waters, as I had learned before going to her, that Jennifer used to be a client of Alice's a few years prior.

    The appointment went wonderful. Jennifer was patient and extremely thorough in her explanation. It was a breath of fresh air. She also used muscle testing to balance out the body's energy with different supplements, but she was very against the liver/gallbladder cleanse. She used different tubes of sample supplements to determine which ones my body needed to help my eye heal. She explained that every person had a field of energy around them. In fact, all objects had an invisible field of energy around them. She used muscle testing to identify how big my field was at that moment. After doing a few demonstrations, she showed me that my field around my body was very weak on my right side. This made sense to me since my right side was where all my problems were located. After going through all the paperwork, I gulped at the price, but I knew I didn't have a choice. Jennifer was sweet, reasonable, and she really had a great approach to this technique. I happily gave over my credit card and we started the process.

I was diligent in taking all of the supplements that she said I needed. Each week, they would change a bit or I would need new ones, as I would start having weird symptoms. Sometimes, I would have strong dizzy spells, stomach aches, and over all I felt swollen and heavy. Each symptom according to Jennifer meant something in the healing process, and we would readjust the supplements as we went along. This was getting a bit expensive since I never knew what my body was going to need next. But, I kept pushing along anyways because I was curious to see how my next scan was.

At my next specialist appointment, four weeks later, I held my scan in my hands. The hole was still about the same size, but at least it hadn't gotten any bigger. All the hard work and nasty tasting drop supplements over the past few weeks had been worth it; since things didn't progress in a negative way. I was hopeful that Jennifer's program had at least gotten the hole to stop growing. After talking with Dr. Stewart, I pushed my next appointment to another four weeks out. I didn't feel comfortable with expanding the time in between visits yet.

I kept seeing Jennifer as often as I could. I was hopeful that this worked, and I figured it would only be time that I needed for the supplements to totally heal my eye. I was so dedicated to this process that I even brought my kids in to have them tested for different

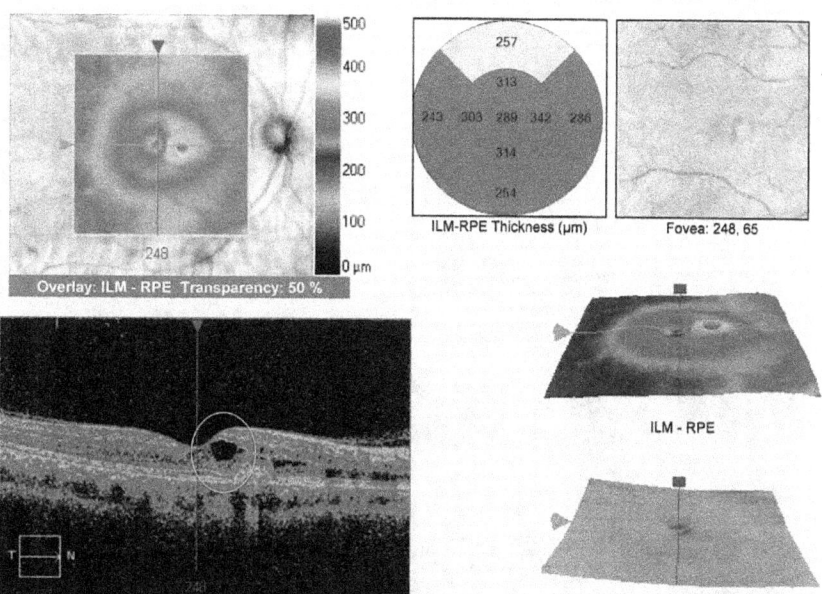

(Photo Caption: OTC Scan shows the hole had improved a small amount from the last appointment.)

things. Dez was still struggling with his breathing from time to time, so I wanted to see that heal as well. It was a lot to juggle when we got home. Every morning and every night I would count out drops and make sure everyone had what they needed. Even Gary went in to try this new approach. He wasn't exactly sold on this idea. His questions were always, "So do you have to take this stuff forever? And how do we travel with all of this? This can't be good to keep doing over and over again. What's in the drops exactly?" I had asked myself the same questions, but I wanted to see if it made an impact on my scans over the next few months. Gary and I didn't completely see eye to eye with it, but he again was willing to support me, since it wasn't doing any harm and was all-natural medicine.

It was now almost one year since my diagnosis. I was pleased with the scan on this visit. I finally saw a hint of improvement. My numbers had dropped just slightly and I felt like I was getting back on track. Dr. Stewart said I still needed an injection, but he was happy to see things stabilizing a bit. I scheduled the next appointment four weeks out and went on my way. I was pleased with

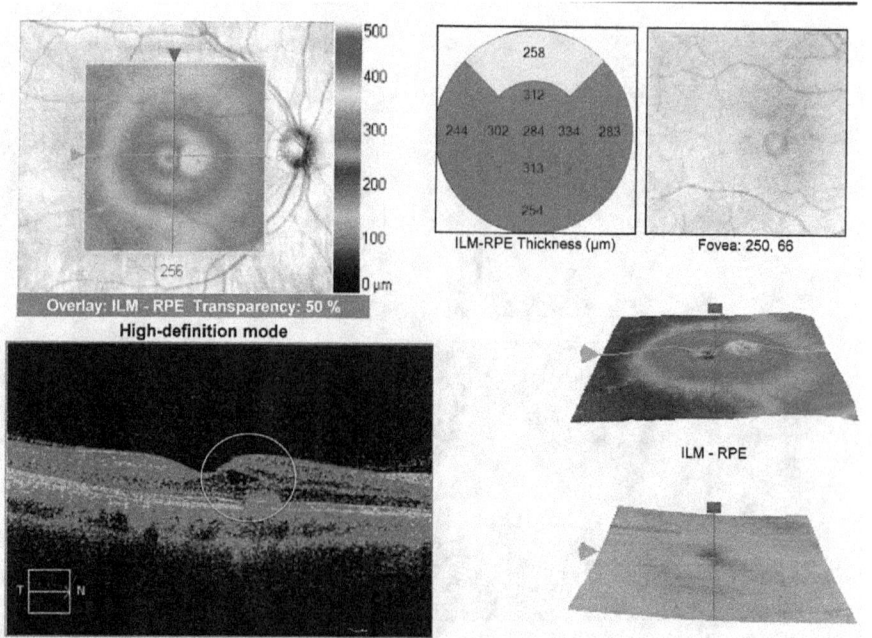

(Photo Caption: OTC Scan taken on 7/5/17 shows a slight improvement from the previous visit.)

the results, but I did wish my results had been a bit more drastic. Yet, I was happy to see my eye was holding strong for now.

I talked to Jennifer right away about my results and she shared in the excitement with me. She also suggested that I travel three hours from home to a town called, Green Bay. Yes, the town of the Green Bay Packers for all of you football-loving fans. The man she wanted me to see was John (name changed for the book). He studied in a type of muscle response testing that helped clear out emotions. She explained that the process might be a little different than what I was used to. Jennifer further explained that she thought there was more going on in my system regarding emotions, and his program would complement her program really well. I knew in my heart that my eye dis-ease was triggered from emotions, so this sounded like another great path to go on. At this point, with two improved specialist appointments under my belt, I was willing to try anything to speed this process up.

My family decided to make a weekend adventure while going to see John. We hadn't traveled at all since we came home from

Clarity

Hawaii. We were all looking forward to getting out of town for the weekend and feeling a bit free. My appointment with John was on a Friday afternoon in July. It was a strange appointment, to say the least. He was a tall, slender man, with a long almost all-gray ponytail. As I sat in the chair across from him, he used muscle testing to see if there was an age in my life that connected the current condition of my eye to an emotional event from the past. This was something that was so foreign to me, but I was excited about it.

    I held my right arm out in front of me so that it was parallel with the ground. He started saying, "Is there an event between ages zero and five that contributed to the state of Nikki's right eye? Is there an event between the ages of five and ten?" This kept going on with different ages and events for over an hour.

    He started picking up on timelines that were affecting my eye in a negative way, and then he would ask what the first thing would be that came to my mind. Immediately, I thought of events. It was as if someone had stuck a picture book in my face and said, "Here you go!" Once we had all the pieces of my past laid out, we figured out what emotions I felt with them. He tested it the same way. My arm would either stay strong against his push or it would drop in total weakness. Finally, he said "Picture the event in your mind as vividly as possible. I'm going to tap on your back in a certain way that will allow the negative energy from the event to process through your system."

    He continued by saying, "This technique can take a long time to fully heal the eye because there are layers upon layers of emotions from experiences in your life that connect to your eye. The buildup of those emotions contributed to your eye misbehaving." He warned me that it might take traveling to Green Bay frequently to work through all of the emotional baggage I had stored up. I decided to see if I felt anything first before committing to this way of thinking. I didn't even fully understand what I was doing yet.

    The process started and as he was tapping I started to see the image in my mind fade away. I fought to get it back, but it was like trying to grab running water. It just slipped away from me. Panicked that I was doing something wrong, I spoke up and told him what was happening. Surprisingly, he assured me that I was doing it right and the treatment was working. Suddenly, the memory was so faint that I could barely recall it. To this day, I still can't honestly bring the memory to the forefront of my mind. This was amazing! Whatever he did literally took away the mental pain of that image.

    I tried to explain to Gary what had happened, but the concept was so out there that it was hard to put into words. Since we were in Green Bay for the weekend, John suggested that I come in on Saturday and do one more session. He was intrigued by my rare case and I could tell he wanted to play a part in solving it. I agreed and the next session was even more impactful than the last. I was sad to leave in a way because I felt like the emotional part was more of my problem than nutrition. I already was eating extremely well, but I was having a hard time controlling the emotional rollercoaster I was on all the time. His program seemed to fit better with my needs and wants than Jennifer's, but the downfall was the distance between us.

    The four weeks had gone by quickly and it was now August 2, 2017. I was thrilled when the nurse brought out my scan and I realized my eye had improved again! I was still going to need an injection since the fluid was obvious, but I was excited that the black hole had gone down quite a bit more from the last time. I felt like I was slowly going in the right direction this time. Although the outcome was still the same, my hope that this would be done soon gave me a little positivity to hang onto.

Clarity

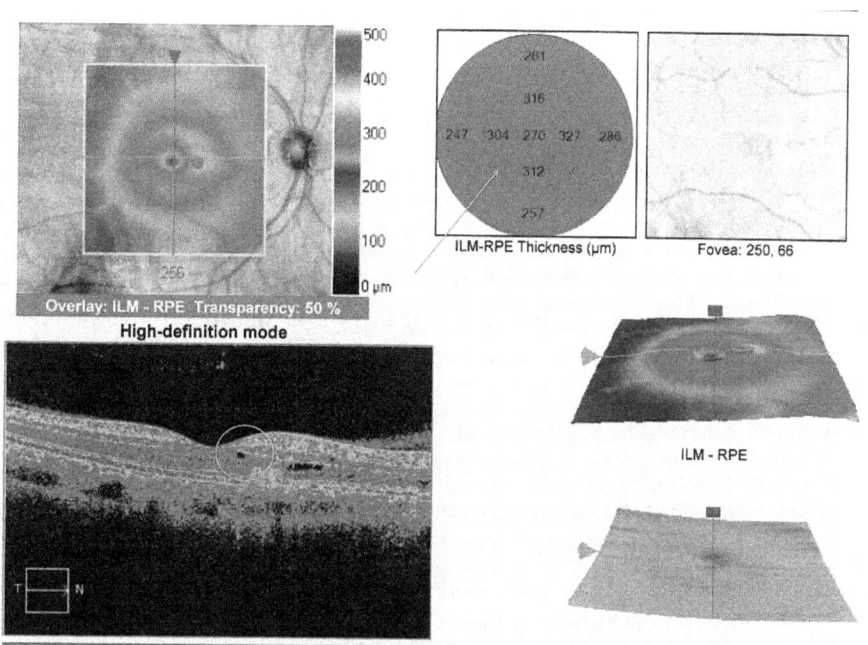

(Photo Caption: OTC Scan taken 8/2/17. The images show another improvement in the numbers since working with Jennifer and John.)

Over the next few months, my scans continued to improve. I saw Jennifer quite frequently to adjust my supplements and continue on the journey. We talked often about my experience with John and how much that seemed to help. She also expressed that she wished she knew how to do that line of work. I agreed with her on how helpful it was, and I was excited to book another session with him. I often wondered if my scan improved because I pushed out some emotional issues from the work that he did. For now though, my scans were starting to slowly move to better results. I was even able to move my appointments out to a full five weeks, and to my amazement they were still getting better. I was hoping to reach a full six weeks again soon. This welcoming progress carried me all the way until December of 2017, and then things took another turn.

WHAT I DID AND WHAT YOU CAN DO: ACTION STEPS 17-20

➤ **Step 17 - Be a Scientist:**

In your healing journey you may be able to play with different parts of your healing routine to test and see if things are getting any better. For me, that was testing out my contacts and seeing if I still needed to have a prism for assistance to clearly see a full image. Maybe you have something like this that gives you a personal calibration other than feelings. Whatever that might be, be brave and try a baby step. Rate how that baby step felt from 1 to 10 in your mind, and possibly write it down in your binder or journal. The more you do this, and test out your baby step in different situations, the more you'll learn about your condition as it effects or maybe does not affect your body in that moment. These little bits of information will help you figure out if you're improving.

A scientist doesn't just look at each of his ideas and say, "Oh well, I guess I'm stuck here forever." No! They go out and test, write notes, and find different ways to test their ideas. For example, I was scared to try my contacts. In my mind, there was no way I would be able to handle having them in my eyes. Because of my circumstances at the time, I didn't have a choice but to try. In doing so, I learned that I could wear my contacts in Hawaii and for some reason not very well in Wisconsin. I didn't figure it out until later, but it gave me hope that my condition could improve and I wasn't doomed to this fate forever. Whatever your situation, choose something to test in a relatively safe manner and try it! See what happens; you might be surprised. When you're testing out your ideas, make sure you make one change at a time. If you do too many at one time, you might not know which one helped or hurt you.

➤ **Step 18 - Remember How Powerful Your Mind Is:**

Your mind is a powerhouse! It has the ability to create, to feel, to analyze, to strategize, to move, to feel pain, and to let go and be happy. Unfortunately, most people don't give much thought to the inner voice that they have and to the powerful mind that allows them to do all the tasks they expect their body to do. Your mind and your emotions, however, are what drive you to be a happy person or an extremely depressed person. For example, my mind was happy and free in Hawaii. I didn't try to control it. I let it be in the state that felt good. As a result, my eye felt great, I could see better, my pain was gone, and I looked younger. All of this was created because of the state of mind I was in. As soon as I started thinking about my stresses back home, the exact opposite happened. Immediately, my eye was a mess and the angry volcano in me let loose.

The point is, give your mind more attention and credit for your condition. There was a quote that was said by Napoleon Hill: "Whatever the mind can conceive and believe, it can achieve." This is so true in any situation. Let's look at my situation again. My mind conceived and believed Hawaii would be a great place of healing, and it was. I was able to wear my contacts like nothing ever happened to my eye. I felt alive and free and, as a result, I didn't have any pain in my body. Now, at the end of the trip, my mind conceived and believed that going home was going to bring me a whole bunch of problems and stresses. My mind soaked up that thought and guess what, it brought me a whole bunch of problems and stresses.

I know sometimes this can be a hard idea to absorb; however, I'm going to take this one step further for you so that you can see how powerful the mind is. In the first part of the story I'm sharing with you, I kept saying and thinking, "Something's going to blow," every time my stress level was reaching a point in me that was causing pure pain and panic. My mind conceived that idea, believed that idea, and the result was a blood vessel literally blowing up in my eye. Was this a coincidence? I don't think so. I looked back at every event that had happened to my family and realized that my stress and worry resulted in the exact thing I was worried about happening!

At this point, you might be thinking, *Okay great, so how do I monitor all these thoughts and feelings inside of my head?* The answer is, you don't. We have millions of thoughts going through the mind all of the time. And that gets to be impossible to manage. If a negative thought or worry enters your mind, recognize it, let it go, and replace it with the exact opposite. In order to do this, you might need to recite the positive idea in your head a few times. Over time, you'll start to form habits of only positive thinking. This will take time and some work, but don't stress over it, just acknowledge it and practice lightly at first.

Now, we can also take this one step further. Your mind works with feelings. It's the feelings that create the events that happen in your life. It's a vibration that's set into motion in the universe. For example, let's go back in the story before I booked the Hawaii trip. I was sitting on my couch in the dead of winter, yet in my mind, I could feel the warm sun and the sand in between my toes. That feeling was large and my mental vibrations made it feel as if I were already there. This is when you know your mind is in the process of conceiving something. Now, you still have to do the physical work, however. I still had to book a trip, and I still had to plan it all. However, when you plant the seed in the brain, and you *feel* what you want to happen, the steps are there to take and they feel easy and effortless.

Your task in this step is to focus on what you want in your healing. What do you truly want? Not your fear, not your worries. This has to be your best positive outcome regarding your healing. I encourage you to take a quiet moment for yourself every day, without distractions, and focus on seeing yourself in the best positive outcome that could come from your healing. Maybe it's seeing your doctor's face and he's saying to you, "YOU'RE HEALED," or maybe it's seeing your son or daughter getting married and, in your body, you feel amazing as you sit and watch them walk down the aisle. Whatever it is, create the picture in your mind every day. Only focus on the positive, because whatever you focus on, your mind will provide that to you in your current life.

➢ **Step 19 - Grow Your Circle:**

Parts of your healing process will feel daunting. This is where your designated cheerleader will really help you keep going on your quest to true health. However, you should also expand your circle to include others in your process as well. For me, I shared my ups and downs with some of our close students in our martial arts school,

Clarity

and a few of the parents at my girls' dance practice. Hearing their words of encouragement or advice really helped me find the right people to help me. They often had a different take on things I could try or they would ask questions that I wouldn't have thought of. It's always a good idea to collaborate with others to help you get an outside view.

My collaboration with others led me to Jennifer. She was an outside person who gave me the tools and knowledge I needed to move forward with my progress. People are amazing if you let them be. You might not jive with everyone you meet on your success path, but you'll learn something each time you collaborate with them. You never know where your path will lead, and, since you're your own scientist on this path, use all the resources you can to heal your condition.

➢ Step 20 - Look into Eastern Medical Techniques:

Jennifer used an Eastern approach to treat my condition. Her process fit well with the Western idea of thinking where you needed to take a medication, in this case a supplement, in order to heal. Although this part lined up in a similar way to my existing thinking, the muscle testing approach was very new to me. I also started to learn how much the mind had an impact on the body through different emotions. My experience with John in Green Bay also gave me a sneak peek into what Eastern medicine was and how it could help without supplements.

Luckily, in this day and age there are quite a few holistic practitioners in the states now who follow along with Eastern medicine philosophies. As much as I believe in the Eastern medicine now, I still believe there's a time and place for Western medicine. For my situation, I needed both types to heal my eye, while I learned what Eastern Medicine was and how powerful the mind is. Hopefully with this book, the learning curve will be shortened for you.

Before you start looking up holistic practitioners, I encourage you to keep reading forward. The rest of my story takes quite a turn and hopefully will lead you to understanding what kind of holistic practitioner to look for if you choose to go that route. I also want to again mention that whatever you do, please still work with your doctor who diagnosed your condition. It's very important to grow your team of healers in all areas. You'll want to make sure you have all the information from all angles so that you can navigate through your condition safely.

** YOUR TO-DO LIST **
17. RESEARCH NEW WAYS TO HEAL THROUGH YOUR OWN TESTS.
18. WRITE DOWN YOUR END GOAL.
19. TELL YOUR STORY TO OTHERS; YOU MIGHT DISCOVER NEW PERSPECTIVES.
20. EXPAND YOUR KNOWLEDGE OF EASTERN MEDICINE.

Chapter 7: Believe

It was December 20, 2017; five weeks since my last really good appointment with Dr. Stewart. I was nervous for my results this time around. I hated to admit it, but I could tell things weren't great in my eye again. Sitting in the musty waiting room, I started testing my eye. I would close my right and look through my left eye, then I would close the left and look out of the right eye. Wavy lines and distorted saran wrap like images greeted my right eye like a pesky reminder of the very first appointment I had. I was beyond frustrated when the nurse brought out my printed results, which showed the ugly black hole was back, and my inflammation had spiked the numbers again. *What in the world?* I thought.

I sat in the semi-comfortable waiting room chair with Gary, and watched the kids play with the toys that were in the corner of the room. Tears rolled down my face as the elderly onlookers showed concern and grace on their faces. I looked at Gary, pretending to ignore the onlookers, and said, "I'm doing everything I can right now. Why is this not working? All of the money I've spent... all of those supplements..." His sad, sympathetic

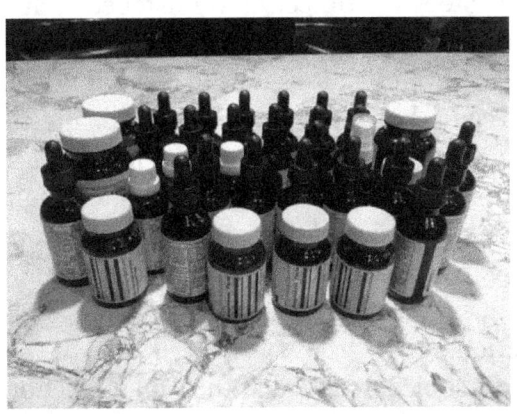

(Photo Caption: Nikki captures a portion of the supplements that she took during this time.)

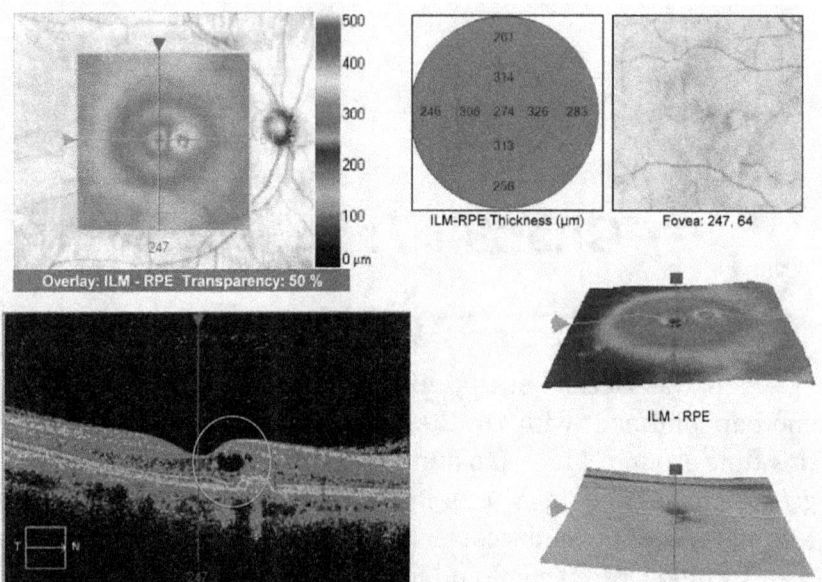

(Photo Caption: OTC Scan shows the fluid is pooling at a faster rate. My numbers have also elevated as well. This is five weeks since an injection.)

look didn't make me feel any better in the moment. He didn't have the answers either as I watched him shake his head left to right in a slow "I don't know" motion.

    Our perplexed conversation was suddenly interrupted when we were called back to Dr. Stewart's office. As we listened to him, my heart fell into my stomach when he suggested that there might be a good chance I'll have to have injections for the rest of my life. I knew this information already, but it didn't sit well with me this time. Dr. Stewart even suggested switching medications, since he was surprised my eye wasn't keeping up on the progress. Changing medications scared me even more, since I thought I was going to die from the throat squeezing experience from the very first shot. A new medication was out of the question at this point. I didn't need to play dare with a different injection.

    Since I didn't have a choice, I agreed to the same injection I had been getting in the past. It had been well over a year already and my body hated getting these injections. Each time I got one now, I could feel the needle busting through scar tissue in my eye from all

Clarity

of the previous injections. It was absolutely the grossest feeling I had ever experienced. Not to mention I still had an issue with my hair falling out and my skin was still not healing. I couldn't get these injections any more, but I couldn't say no to them either. I was on a rotating cycle that I couldn't jump out of.

I immediately texted Jennifer about what I had just learned. My frustrated feelings just got a hard shove into overdrive, and were now reading terrified on my emotion meter. I needed something, anything, that made sense right now, and I was hoping her words would present that to me. Unfortunately, Jennifer's words did the opposite of that.

Her message back was just as unsure as I was at this point. I could tell that she didn't have the answers either. Her main fear was also the injections and what they did in my body. She wanted to test me after I had an injection to see how strong my energy field was and then compare that to before I had the injection. I thought this was a good idea, but I wasn't sure how it was going to help the situation that I was currently in.

I also suggested to her that I started juicing veggies and fruits heavily again a few weeks before this appointment. Since it was early winter, I was trying to bump up my immune system, so I picked up an old but good habit again. The problem was, every time I juiced I would get a stabbing pain in my skull. It almost felt like I had ten, tight pony tail holders in my hair, just squeezing all of my hair follicles to the point of pain. This was a common complaint I had when I first started with Jennifer, but, unfortunately, we never got to the bottom of why it was happening.

After frantically reviewing my scans and the dates over the next few weeks, I realized a connection in my scans and when I was juicing. I was heavily juicing right before we went to Hawaii and now I was juicing the same way and my OCT scan numbers were very similar. I also realized I literally lost eight months of progress in one tiny appointment. I still hadn't really put all the pieces together yet when my next appointment with Dr. Stewart popped up on my calendar. I had pushed it out to five weeks again in hopes that a miracle would happen and my numbers would be better. Although I tried to stay optimistic, the next five weeks were long and excruciating in the pain department both physically and mentally. I again knew as I walked into the clinic that the results were going to be bad. My juvenile eye switching test showed again those terrifying wavy lines.

Unfortunately, my simplistic eye test was telling the truth. I again needed another shot and badly. My scan was even worse than the last. Dr. Stewart suggested that I needed to get the injections closer together now. He now recommended every two to four weeks. I was crushed, defeated, and I felt like my heart was pulled out of my chest and trampled on. My husband and children looked at me with love and compassion, mixed with a little fear. They were there for me with hugs and showers of kisses after Dr. Stewart left the room. I was starting to go into a fast spiral slump as I sat in the examination chair, staring at the scan of the ugly black mess. My reality and my belief that I could heal this disease were butting heads like two mighty-male rams.

Before I left Dr. Stewart's office, I asked for the ingredients that were listed on the packaging of the injection. I was hoping Jennifer could test each one of those ingredients to see how badly they affected me. The only problem was the office didn't have a full list of them, and honestly, what did it matter what ingredients were in the injections if I still had to receive them in order to save my sight. I couldn't treat these injections like they were an allergy food and stay away from it. After sending Jennifer a new message about my current state, I reread her replied messages again from my last December appointment and awaited her reply. I was reminded again from that message, that she didn't have the answers. When her new message popped up in response to my current bad news with only a "sounds good," I knew I was in trouble. I was on a hamster wheel and it was spinning at an uncontrollable rate. I knew it, and Jennifer knew it. As much as both of us wanted the answers, we didn't have them.

Since my eye journey had been so long and daunting, most of the families in our martial arts school knew my situation. It was pretty obvious when I went to work with my eye looking like a swollen mess after an injection. One evening after the latest devastating appointment with Dr. Stewart, a parent came up to me to talk and see how I was doing. She suggested that I go across the street to a man named Dr. Khan. She claimed that he could really help me.

I knew the name from hearing he was a great chiropractor in town. I was confused as to why she thought a chiropractor could help my eye. And to be honest, after my last experience with a chiropractor, it was the last thing I wanted to do. She rambled on and explained her urgent push, "Oh, he's great! He does what Jennifer does, but there aren't any supplements. The muscle testing he does just clears out the issues. He can even help with food allergies. You can just clear it out and then eat the food without problems." I looked at her with wide saucer eyes. "REALLY?!" I knew she had mentioned his name to me a few times over the months while I had been seeing Jennifer, but I never asked questions to learn more. My assumption was that he was only a chiropractor. In reality, he had a tool that I desperately needed.

The next day, I booked an appointment and surprisingly, I could get in within a few days of calling. Was it possible that my belief was still alive? Could this be too good to be true? The questions start flooding me as I prepared myself for the

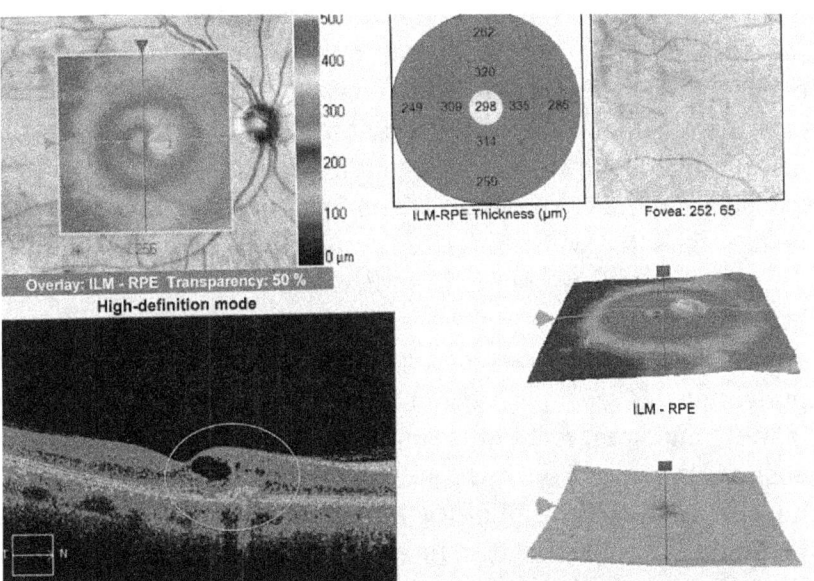

(Photo Caption: OCT Scan taken 1/24/18. The fluid has increased since the last image.)

appointment. I was nervous, excited, and determined to fix this. I again didn't know anything about this approach, but I felt confident that I could gain some major progress based on my last few years. Reluctantly, I approached Gary again and explained my plan. He surprised me with his unwavering support. We had a long conversation and we both agreed that I had to keep on searching. The injection wasn't the solution. The answers were somewhere else and I had to keep looking. I knew there was something to the muscle testing that was working based on my results fluctuating, but there were holes in the approach that I currently was on. I also knew that my body wasn't really healing, since I still had all of my other symptoms to some degree. It was time for a change.

January 31, 2018, just one week since my devastating news from Dr. Stewart that he wanted my injections closer together, I walked into an updated older building to see Dr. Khan. The building had been an old bank and was now turned into remodeled office spaces. Dr. Khan's Office was on the upper level. I walked in, not knowing what to expect. I hadn't been in this place since I was a kid. Quick visions of me running to get a sucker from the teller window flashed in my mind. To my surprise, it looked exactly as it did back then with the teller windows still in place, the furniture hadn't moved, and the vault door sat quietly open. It was a weird comfortable feeling as I walked through the doors, yet I felt extremely nervous about my appointment. The tug-of-war on my heart made me hover for a moment at the bottom of the stairs as I looked around. I gathered myself and proceeded to follow my belief up the stairs that whispered, "This way. This is your answer." I took a breath, opened the door to the office, and stepped inside to test my bravery once again.

This office was simple, not over the top, and very professional. The employees were extremely polite and I felt comfort in watching them work with each other as I waited to be called back. Soon my thoughts were interrupted by Dr. Khan himself introducing himself. He was in his mid-30s with dark hair and a friendly smile. I assumed he would have an Indian accent with his last name being Khan. I was surprised when he spoke; he didn't have an accent at all. I followed him back to the patient room with nerves dancing

Clarity

around my stomach. He sat across from me as I sat in the chair next to the wall. The room smelled of fresh orange cleaner and was filled with a natural sunlight glow from the winter sun. It was calming and it helped my nerves loosen their grip on my stomach just a bit.

I boldly started my story about why I was there to see him. I decided to go into this appointment extremely forthcoming. He needed to know how serious I was about healing and I didn't have time to waste. I even looked at him and said, "No offense to chiropractic work, but I had a horrible experience and I don't want to be cracked ever again. But, I am very interested in the other work that you do." He didn't seem offended at all by my bold statement, which was a good sign for me. He continued to ask questions about my history and all the symptoms I was experiencing. He said the protocol that he used was called NAET™. The acronym stands for Nambudripad's Allergy Elimination Techniques, which was invented by Dr. Devi Nambudripad. I was intrigued when he used the word allergy elimination. I wasn't sure if this would work for me, since I wasn't allergic to anything that I knew of. However, if he could eliminate allergies, could this help eliminate my issues with food and the injections? "It would be nice to get rid of the elephant baby belly and the cold-like symptoms after an injection," I expressed to him.

Intrigued, I listened harder to the words that he said next. "This technique uses acupressure to allow the energy to flow better through the Chinese meridian lines. When we do the technique, we can look into seven different groups that can become allergies to the body. They are food, chemicals, emotions, events, concepts, people, and behaviors. We will use muscle testing to help us narrow down what you're allergic to." He continued, "The best way I can explain this is if I show you. Do you mind laying on the table? I'll test and see if NAET will even work on healing your food issues, and I'll also test to see if it will work on helping the healing process for your right eye." My mind was already jumping in excitement. I couldn't believe all of these things could be tested with muscle testing! And I couldn't believe people could be allergic to all of the things he stated. I was excited! My heart was racing in hopes that the testing would show that I had a new path. It was either this, or beat my head against a wall, since I didn't have any other options.

Just as in the last few practices that I visited, I lay on the table, lifted my right arm in the air, and the muscle testing began. He was gentle, yet applied the correct pressure as he pushed my arm down towards my hip. As he did this, he showed me a question and response technique writing yes or no questions on pieces of paper. He placed a small piece of paper in my hand without telling me what it said and tested my arm. Then he showed me the paper afterwards. I was blown away. The paper read, "Is your name Nikki?" My arm had gone weak, indicating a yes. He showed me the other paper which said, "Are you wearing purple pants?" My arm had stayed strong, which indicated a no. This was also correct, since I had black pants on. Then he proceeded by showing me that you can ask the question out loud as well as writing it down and he could get the same results. I was astonished! Then he asked out loud the most important question, "Can NAET help the healing process in Nikki's right eye." He pushed on my arm and I tried with all my might to hold it up. There wasn't any strength in my arm and it fell to my hip. I couldn't remember which way my arm should go for no when asking a question, so I looked at him in a moment of panic. He kindly looked back and said, "It looks like it will help."

I was trying to hold my excitement in, but I suddenly blurted out, "Oh thank goodness!" We kept testing all seven categories to see where my body was at. In one appointment, I found out that I was allergic to quite a bit of the food I was eating, and I had multiple events that contributed to my condition. I also had allergies to certain chemicals, environmental things, and people. All sorts of combinations were coming to my mind and I quickly realized so many aspects of my life were connected to the contribution of my eye misbehaving. I shook my head in amazement and looked at him, "So we can use pressure points, reverse the effect these things have on my body, and then I won't have an issue with them anymore?" He answered back, "Yes, but you have to be prepared that this could take quite some time. Some of these things could be interconnected quite a bit. It all depends on how your body does with clearing them and we won't know that until we start. Some people it takes only a

Clarity

few appointments, and others have a tangle of items to clear and it can take months."

I immediately told him I was in! Shortly afterwards, we tested all of the supplements that I had been taking from Jennifer's program. We found out that since I was allergic to things like Vitamin A, Vitamin C, etc., all of the supplements and the juicing I had been doing were actually harming my body more. Plus, most of the supplements I was taking didn't seem to help my eye in the healing process either, according to his tests. I felt conflicted because I had followed Jennifer's program for so long and was dedicated to it. But Dr. Khan's results explained everything that I had questioned and struggled with before!

My increasing head pain after juicing, my eye scans getting worse, and my body just overall not healing was all explained in an hour appointment. How could my body heal if I was allergic to so many things? Especially, the vitamins. No matter how hard I worked to keep up with good nutrition, my body was rejecting it. I knew it was true from looking over my detective notes over the last few years. Without having the ability to absorb good nutrition, my body was breaking down from being starved from what it truly needed to heal. I couldn't wait to start his program and I was so ready to fix this once and for all. No band aids any more, just helping the body do what it does best, heal!

The one question that I had was, "How in the world did I become allergic to all of these things." Dr. Khan sent me a video that helped further explain how NAET works. As I watched, everything started to click for me. The video basically explains that NAET comes from a background of the following practices: "Acupuncture, Allopathy, Chiropractic, Nutritional Therapy, and Kinesiology."

When a person has a traumatic experience and when the body is in shock, anything that is exposed to it in that timeframe can become an allergy. So the human body's energy field and the field of each of those items can repel each other, which then results in an allergic reaction. It's the body's way of putting up its protection walls with an immune response of possible cold-like symptoms, aches and pains, etc. When you use the NAET treatment, acupressure is applied to certain spots along the spine, while holding a test tube or word of that allergen in your hand. This specific technique will help the flow of energy in the body and will teach the body to let go of the immune response to the specific allergen.[13] I've added the link of the video on my website at www.nikkiengels.com/naet for you.

This new information was a game changer for me! I had had multiple events of trauma in my life, like Dez being in the N.I.C.U, the house fire, the accumulation of the business struggles, and the unfortunate negative chiropractic appointment that led to my problems. All of my doctors, including our family practitioner, didn't have the answers to why my body was having some of the weirdest symptoms.

Over the last year of searching for the answer, I also had a regular allergy test done and blood work drawn. The results turned up empty. NAET testing took a different approach to allergies. Dr. Khan was testing energetically if I had allergies to certain things. Some of these allergies, for example, having a true allergy to a person or a person's behavior, couldn't be tested with a traditional blood test. This was phenomenal news for me. This knowledge explained why I had constant pain in some parts of my body, and why other pain, like feeling a squeeze of ten tight ponytails in my hair, would come and go. My symptoms were happening based on the allergy that I was or wasn't being exposed to at that time.

After watching the video and sitting back and thinking about all of the events, emotions, and people that were connected in my life, I knew NAET could help. Things were starting to make more sense and my belief was now in the driver's seat; I was happy, excited, and ready to take action! I knew I was a tangled mess of emotions and trauma that we were going to have to fix, but I finally had the clarity I was looking for.

Pushing aside the thought on how my body could heal itself through NAET, I asked a different question now. How was it that my body could read the words on that paper Dr. Khan had put in my hand, and how did my body know the correct answer? I went back to my thoughts about the book I saw on the study of water back in college that I had seen in the library. The image of that book danced in my mind as I thought about NAET more. Could this all tie together? I immediately ordered the book, *The Hidden Messages in*

Clarity

Water by Dr. Masaru Emoto, and dove into how this could even be possible. The research was astonishing and my belief had brought me the knowledge that I needed to move forward in my healing again.

WHAT I DID AND WHAT YOU CAN DO: ACTION STEPS 21-24

➢ **Step 21 - Review Your Progress:**

There will be points in your healing journey when you'll want to step back and review where you are. It's important to do this in a healthy amount of time. You'll want to give each process time to work, but you don't want to be stuck in it for too long if your results aren't helping your progress. For me, I struggled with this idea because I'm a loyal person to good people. Jennifer was that person to me and I didn't want to hurt her feelings. There came a point, though, when I had to pick my health and my healing as the first priority and not someone else's feelings.

If you're a person who will do more for others than you'll do for yourself, this part can be very challenging for you. It's important to use your journal and your binder to help you navigate through this section. If you've tried different approaches of healing with an outside team, most likely, you'll feel like you have established a relationship with these people. Remember, it's okay to be honest with them and tell them how you're feeling about your progress. If you aren't getting the results that you believe you can get, then it's time to talk to them and or find a new path. Most likely when you feel like you're up against a wall, there's a new path awaiting you. You just have to be brave, look for it, and take it.

My last piece of advice on this section is to watch out for any practice or person who keeps you unhealthy on purpose just so they can make more money from you. Unfortunately, we live in a world that thrives on money rather than the good of the person. You may also have a great person, but their scope of practice is only limited to what they know. For example, Jennifer is a great person, but her training wasn't able to get to the root cause of my issues, which happened to be emotional trauma. She didn't know that I was going around in circles in my healing progress because she didn't have the training in emotional healing to help. So, in a situation like this, it's a good idea to try things, but also be your own judge and find different resources and ways of thinking. Stay open, ask your team lots of questions, but, most importantly, listen to your heart and listen to what path you should take.

> **Step 22 - Keep Believing:**

Belief is one of the most important aspects in your healing journey. Ask yourself right now, do you believe you can heal? Hopefully, your answer is a resounding YES! If it is, build on this and allow it to grow. I will give you some steps on how to make this more powerful as you read on.

If your answer is no or maybe you said yes but you can feel the doubt behind your answer, then here is your first step. Each day, write down the words, "I am healed," or write "My (list your body part) is fully healed. At first, you're most likely going to feel like this is a joke or your lying to yourself. But once you form the habit of writing this affirmation, (a habit takes 21 days to form), you'll start to feel the new belief taking over. This is a great tool on how you can anchor a positive belief over a negative one.

Another step is going to be battling other's beliefs against your own. This is a difficult part because most of us really value other's opinions over our own. The trick that I used to keep my belief alive was any time my doctors or friends would cast doubt, I would simply say, "I hear you, but I AM figuring this out." That was enough to have them understand that I was serious about my healing, and I didn't want to be told that my condition was the end of me. Surprisingly, taking this stance actually helped them start to root for me as well. They wanted to see me succeed. Maybe some truly wanted it, and maybe others wanted me to succeed so that they could stop hearing about my ups and downs. Either way, their positivity helped, but it took my concrete view and belief that I wasn't going to stop until I was fully healed. Keeping that power burning inside allows your mind to start accessing what it needs to heal, and the paths you need to take will start to open. The bottom line is, you have to *feel* and *believe* with all of your heart that *you're healing*.

Clarity

Even if your answer is a resounding yes, you might battle moments of doubt. After all, we're human and your mind will wander to the darker side from time to time. If it does, pull out your journal and start writing your affirmations down of what exactly you want. Do this a few times, then call or talk to your cheerleader and ask them for a pep talk. Your job in this moment of doubt is to get your thoughts back on track. Once you feel steady, take a deep breath and know that you're okay!

➢ **Step 23 - Study Water:**

I mentioned in my story that I read a book called *The Hidden Messages in Water*. The book is written and based on the Japanese scientist, Dr. Masaru Emoto's work. The author thoroughly discusses his lab results of how showing water different words can develop different crystals when frozen. As he shows his studies throughout the book, both visually and verbally, the author paints a great picture of how our positive or negative thoughts can affect our inner body in a physical way, since our bodies are made up mostly of water. This book offered a few interesting revelations for me about healing.[14]

Thinking back to my patch and the word *Clarity* neatly glued on with crystals, I now understood why this word was so impactful and important. I was gaining clarity in all areas of health. Even though I, at the time, wasn't healed all the way, I was learning a lot about my condition and my strength inside. I understood, from Dr. Emoto's work, that there was more going on in my body than just a disease. There was a reason for this and it was the fact that I kept repeating to myself and to others that, "something was going to blow." My body felt and heard me say that phrase over and over again, and when the stress became too much, the blood vessel blew. This was an impactful moment when I realized that my words, my stress, and my trauma where all tied to creating this condition. Realizing how important words really are, I made a bracelet that I wear every day that says, "Right Eye Healed." This bracelet is not only read by my body, but it is a constant reminder of the path I'm on. If I was having a bad day, I would look down and read my bracelet to become more centered. Now that I could see scientific proof that words are powerful, it allowed me to believe even more that I could heal my condition.

How does all of this apply to you? My first suggestion would be to read the book *The Hidden Messages in Water*. This will fully explain why it's so important to speak kindly to yourself and to others. Once you understand the studies that took place, it will be easier for you to understand how words can change the way the cells in your body react and how, if given the right words, your body can start to heal. I would also suggest holding a piece of paper that states what you want healed a few times throughout the day, or make a bracelet like I did. The only rule here is whatever you write has to read in the past tense.

For example, "My right eye is healed" is the correct way, rather than "My right eye is healing." Make sure to use words that state it already happened. This will allow your body to read it and think, *Oh, this has already happened, I better catch up and it should be healed.* If you put the words as healing, your progress will be just that; healing, but you'll never fully get to the state of healed. Overall, be careful of the words you choose to write and the words you use in your speech every day. Think of your words being reflected back inward as you say them. I bet if you pictured a mirror and every word you said bounced off the mirror and then went into your heart, you'd be a lot more careful about the language you used.

> **Step 24 - Visualize and Write on the Wall:**

In Step 18, I talked about how your mind can create whatever you feel. This is important when you're thinking and feeling about your own condition. Once you've worked through all of the grief and frustration with your condition, let your belief take over. Really feel like you're totally healed, or a better way to understand this, is to imagine the way you will feel when your doctor tells you that you're fully healed. In order for you to attract healing into your life, you have to *feel* the feelings as if you're already at that point.

For me, sitting down and visualizing was a really difficult task to complete. Being a wife, a mom of three, plus having a dog, and the constant reminder of work from my cell phone pinging all day, was far from the best setup to start to visualize what I wanted

Clarity

for myself. The thought actually became a chore in my mind. Until one day, I was again thinking about how the water studies related to visualization. I had the solution on how to visualize better in the shower, as I watched the steam turn into beads of possibility. If water could read words, they must also read emotions. I started to write on the glass wall of our shower "My right eye is healed." I closed my eyes and imagined that each droplet of water could read those words and in turn would send my message out into the world. Suddenly, I realized that I could surely take a few moments of my showers to re-center my thoughts for the day and focus my intentions on what I truly wanted. It was the only time and place I could find in my busy life that I could allow my mind to travel to all the positive possibilities.

Your task for this step is to find your place of relaxation for your daily visualization. Your place doesn't have to be the shower. This just happened to be where I felt the most relaxed, and quite honestly, where all the distractions were put on hold for a few minutes. I recommend finding a space each day where you can put away all the distractions and concentrate only on you. So, for the sake of this step, I will lead you through a guided visualization.

Imagine you're sitting in your garden, flowers all around you, and you can hear a quiet stream flowing nearby. As you sit, you start to take notice of all the beauty and sounds around you. You become more and more comfortable and relaxed as you take in a few deep breaths. Slowly, you start to close your eyes. At first you might see darkness as your eyelids cover your beautiful eyes. Then slowly, the image starts to appear. You're in your doctor's office. You look down at your hands and see they are calm and stable. You feel your heartbeat and it is beating at an exciting rate. Today is the day that you know you're healed. Today is the day that your doctor is going to confirm what you already know and feel.

For some reason you need to hear your doctor say the words to have it fully sink in. The doctor opens the door and you feel excited for the first time. He enters the room with a big smile and greets you like an old friend as he shakes your hand. He takes a quiet look at your results, does a quick examination, and then sits back. Your heart races a little more, your emotions start to activate in your throat, and you realize you're holding your breath. He opens his mouth and lets out the words, "Congratulations, you're healed!" The breath you've been holding onto suddenly shoots out of your mouth and you're flooded with joy and happiness throughout your entire body. You did it! You healed yourself, and your hard work was worth it.

Sit in this marvelous moment for as long as you'd like. Take it all in and add on to the story if you so choose. When you're ready, slowly start to wiggle your fingertips until you feel yourself back in your relaxing space. Slowly start to open your eyes, and smile with the mental journey you just allowed yourself to discover. Do this visualization at least once a day, then take action to heal yourself.

** YOUR TO-DO LIST **

21. ASSESS YOUR PROGRESS AND DECIDE IF YOU NEED TO MAKE CHANGES.
22. KNOW AND TRUST YOUR NEW POSITIVE BELIEF.
23. READ THE BOOK *THE HIDDEN MESSAGES IN WATER*, BY DR. MASARU EMOTO.
24. VISUALIZE EVERY DAY ON YOUR DOCTOR TELLING YOU THAT YOU'RE HEALED.

Chapter 8: Love and Yoga

The next few weeks working with Dr. Khan were exciting yet challenging. We only had three weeks to work together on my case before my next specialist appointment. I was determined to skip an injection so my effort was beyond one hundred percent. We first started with the food category. Dr. Khan suggested that this would be a good place to start so that we could reteach my energy lines to look at healthy, organic foods as a positive healing tool, rather than an allergy. As we started the process, it became clear to me that all of the foods that gave me trouble were all linked to my eye. The right eye had a line of energy that ran down the back of my head, through the liver, and into my pinky toe on my right foot. In my body, this line of energy was blocked, which didn't allow for the flow of energy to correctly reach my right eye. Without the proper flow of energy, my right eye malfunctioned. This protocol allowed these lines of energy to open up and flow the way they were intended to.

As we did the treatments, my body would flair up an allergy response. This was the most challenging aspect of NAET; however, I welcomed the symptoms. It was comforting to know that when I felt something strange and weird within my body, that it was the energy lines clearing out the negative response. One by one, my body was pushing out the allergy to foods and I was able to start testing this protocol.

As soon as I was done clearing wheat, I went to my favorite restaurant with my sister Karlie to put it to the test. I hadn't been able to eat at restaurants in some time, since most of them didn't have gluten free options. I ordered a hollandaise egg sandwich. My taste buds were dancing in excitement, but my stomach was nervous to try and eat the English muffin. I finished about half of my meal, and as I was talking to my sister, I suddenly realized that my stomach was perfectly fine. It didn't hurt and it wasn't extended like it usually would be after eating this meal. I was ecstatic! The first test worked and I was thrilled to know that at least my stomach would be better. This also gave me hope that my eye would heal as well.

My specialist appointment was coming up very soon, and unfortunately my eye was acting like a storm was brewing deep within. I really didn't want to have another injection, but I didn't have enough time with the NAET protocol to skip an injection. Dr. Khan and I both felt that we were going to have to let my body call the shots on when I would need an injection. And after the injection happened, we would use the NAET protocol to balance out my body to help it process the injection better. I was curious about how I would feel after doing a "brain body balance" clearing after the injection and also clearing the medication itself. I needed desperately to feel better after these injections, because quite honestly, I felt like walking death when that medication was in my system. Even if the clearing allowed my body to feel better by ten percent, I'd take it.

It was now the end of February in 2018, only four weeks and five days since my last visit with Dr. Stewart. I dreaded going back in to face the frustrating news that I could predict beforehand. The negative truth coming from Dr. Stewart always made the situation seem more concrete and real. This appointment wasn't any different. Dr. Stewart looked at the scans with me and said it looked very similar to four weeks ago. His recommendation of course was another injection or aka invasion of my eye at this point. He also recommended that I be seen every four to six weeks based on how bad my scans were. He didn't feel comfortable pushing out my injections any farther than that. Surprisingly, I wasn't as devastated as I had been in the past, since I was able to avoid his previous advice on getting an injection every two to four weeks.

I felt a sense of relief that I found Dr. Khan and the NAET protocol to help me with this. Pivoting in a new direction for my healing gave me a confidence that I hadn't had in a long time. I received another shot and decided to push Dr. Stewart's advice by booking my next appointment to a full six weeks. This was a bold move on my part because the last few months I felt the need for an injection at about week four or sooner. Not only was I taking a leap of faith in NAET, but I was also testing my inner strength. I didn't know how much pain I was going to be in, trying to get to six weeks, but I also knew I had to give my body a fighting chance to show me it could heal.

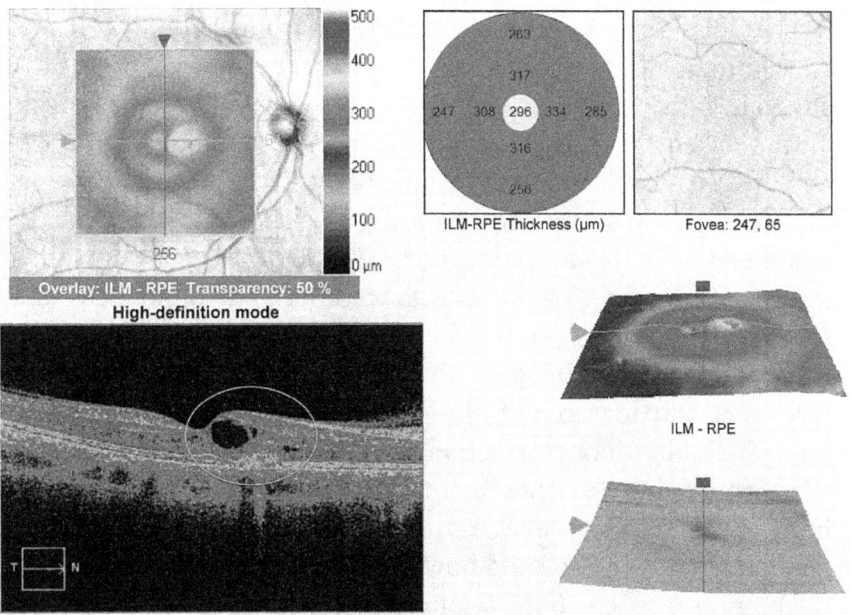

(Photo Caption: OCT Scan taken 2/26/18. The image shows that at 4 weeks and five days the fluid is about the same as the previous appointment.)

Dr. Khan and I diligently kept working through the items that I was allergic too. One by one, we worked through all the foods, chemical, and environmental aspects that my body wasn't processing well. Sometimes, we had to go back and relink a food to one of the new allergies I was working on. It wasn't always as easy as clearing wheat and then always being okay with it. My body was a tangled mess of allergies. It had stored an allergy response in multiple ways to wheat and other things. Even though I cleared it on its own and I didn't have a reaction that day in the restaurant, didn't mean I cleared wheat fully yet. This pesky little wheat energy and a few other foods were also tangled in with certain chemicals I was exposed to. Dr. Khan and I had to put the two items together and clear it that way. It sounds like a difficult and daunting task, but while I was doing it, I felt a million times better after I cleared it. It didn't matter how many ways things were connected, I could physically feel healthier from pushing out a new combination. I welcomed all the new combination groups we did, and I was starting to learn how to listen to my body as symptoms would pop up.

All of the new information I was learning about NAET really started to open my eyes on how the body processes energy, how it stores negative emotions, and how it has the ability to heal itself. I always asked Dr. Stewart about the medication going into my eye and how that could affect my whole body. To him, this didn't make any sense because the medication was going into the eyeball, a contained unit inside of the body. He didn't feel as though the medication would have any effects on other parts of my body at all. It would and should only affect the eye. I knew this wasn't true because I felt the walking death hit me after every injection. NAET now was starting to put the pieces together for me. Western medicine didn't look at the body, mind, and emotions as a whole. Western medicine teaches doctors to look at the malfunction in the body at the physical level, rather than looking at the mind/body being connected as one and how the energy flows or doesn't flow in the body as it reacts to the malfunction.

Interestingly, while going through the allergy connections my body put together, I saw a direct link to my emotional state and the malfunctioning of the eye and how it would present itself. Looking over my doctor's notes from this period, he documents that I said multiple times how stress seemed to bring on pain under my eye and black floaters were popping up during events of stress. In my heart, I always felt as though stress was a rather large component to why my body was violently reacting the way it had been over the years. Since learning more about NAET and how important energy flows were, I decided to expand my knowledge and try to support the work I was doing through NAET by adding yoga to calm my stress.

Clarity

I didn't know much about yoga other than seeing some fancy poses on the Internet. I had been teaching fast-paced fitness classes for years, so the thought of slowing down and learning an art that was all about relaxing seemed foreign to me. However, I was all about flipping my perspectives in order to keep growing and moving along with the healing progress. Over the next few weeks, I kept up with my appointments with Dr. Khan, which were three times a week, and allowed him to use NAET to heal the blockages as well as some noncracking chiropractic techniques to loosen up the pain in my neck and right back/hip area. These areas would become sore or tight as we worked out the allergies that were connected to those meridian lines. It became clear to me, while doing the NAET protocols, that the pain I had felt for so long in my back/side area was directly connected to my liver channel, which ran up to my right eye. When I cleared an event, I would feel that area become sore again. So, the chiropractic work helped keep my body loose enough to gain some comfort while clearing the issue we were working on at the time.

In alignment to working on the physical healing, I decided to research yoga schools and become certified to hopefully help move along the emotional healing quicker. I didn't want to just take yoga classes; I wanted to understand it at a deeper level. The problem was, when I looked up how to get certified, I couldn't find anything in my area. Every program suggested traveling for a few weeks to a remote location in a tropical place. This sounded lovely, don't get me wrong. But the thought of leaving my family, traveling alone, and doing something out of my comfort zone with my eye the way it was, sounded like it would only hurt my emotional state more than help it. Yet, I felt this urge to learn this art. I kept digging and by chance, I ended up finding a school that was only an hour away. They specialized in a style of yoga called Viniyoga™.

I was intrigued by the school because it sounded like it lined up with what my body needed at the time. They worked on breathing techniques and concentrated on matching the breath to the movements of the practice. This allowed the body to relax into postures, rather than force the body to stay in a posture for a long time, like some other yoga styles suggested. Viniyoga™ was a more relaxing and therapeutic concept to allow the body to heal and rebuild from the inside out.

After reading more on the yearlong commitment, I decided to apply even though the application process had already closed. Luckily, the teachers liked my story and I was accepted into the program. My first assignment in the program was to study other yoga schools. I was instructed to take a few classes and journal on my experience with them. This sounded like a fun task and it just so happened to again line up with my next big growing step forward.

Gary and I decided to take another trip to Hawaii at the end of April where I would start my training. This was important to the both of us, because we wanted to test out my eye in this magical place again. I also felt it was important to take my training in a place that brought me the most peace and ease. My appointment with Dr. Stewart fell perfectly in line with our travel dates and I was able to see him a few weeks before we left. To my amazement the results were quite pleasing since I was able to see less fluid in the eye. Not only was there less fluid, but I was reminded that I had pushed my

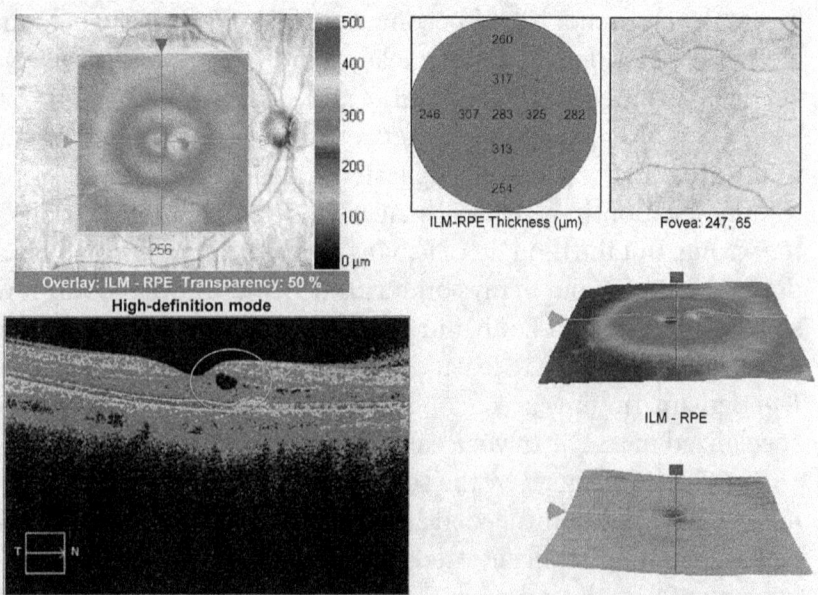

(Photo Caption: The OTC Scan taken 4/9/17 shows after pushing out the appointment to a full six weeks, the fluid has decreased even though there was more time put in between appointments.)

appointment out to a full six weeks. I hadn't been able to do this since March of 2017; a whole year ago. I received my 19th injection on April 9, 2018, a few weeks prior to leaving. Since the hole and fluid were still pretty large, I needed to have security before we left for our trip, so an injection was necessary.

The trip was as magical as the first. I found myself able to wear my contacts most of the trip without any problems. My vision was stable and I didn't seem to have as many issues with things like pressure changes in the planes. I was beyond excited to also notice that I wasn't having as many problems with food on this trip compared to the last trip. So far, NAET had been proven to work quite well. Before I left, we also discovered that I needed to clear my allergy to radiation and changes in temperature. This allergy explained why the first trip caused my dizzy spell on the plane. Since I arrived in Hawaii without the same negative effects as the first time, I felt my confidence soar with my healing progress.

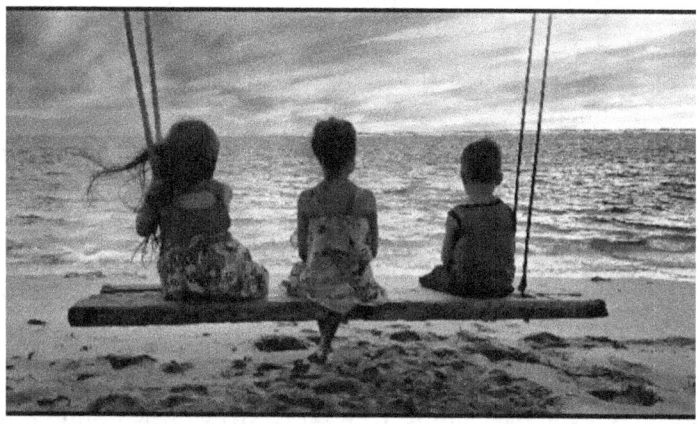

(Photo Caption: The Engels' children looking at the ocean while sitting on a homemade driftwood swing. Photo taken by Gary Engels.)

With my newfound confidence, I began to understand at a deeper level why I pushed so hard to make this trip happen. I first wanted to confirm my positive progress with NAET.™ I also had to find out if I had somehow imagined all the great things that happened to me on the first trip to Hawaii, or if what I experienced really did happen. The interesting thing was, the more I understood energy work, the more I realized that I truly felt magic, or a high energy vibration in Hawaii. The island was charged with lots of positive energy from the ocean, sun, volcanic land, and positive people. The more I paid attention, the more I absorbed the positive energy, and it was healing me. Reflecting further, I had to make this trip because it was important for me to break up the stress that the winter months brought for our family. Our winters were long in northern Wisconsin, and we worked hard throughout them. Come spring, we all needed a break, and I needed to be recharged from the wonderful, magical energy that's stored in Hawaii.

I often heard people say, "Make sure you love yourself," through stressful times in life. I never knew what that meant exactly. While on this trip, I sat on the beach one evening, the family was running around in the sand and playing on a makeshift driftwood swing, and I thought about this saying. Then it hit me, this trip was about loving myself. It was about letting go of all of the negative stresses and letting myself truly relax. I needed to be here to test my theory of this magical place. I needed to stop and recharge my batteries. I had to take this time so that I could be the best wife, mom, and business owner that I could be.

There was so much growth that took place within me while being on this island, that I realized this was me loving myself. This is what that quote meant. Take the time to do what makes you feel amazingly happy. Loving yourself truly meant, letting your stress go, be wild and free, and let your heart sing as loud as it wanted to. This was so hard for me to do because other's expectations of me often made me feel like I had to live in a box. But here, on this island, I could be whoever I wanted to be. My stress was gone, and I could fully concentrate on listening to my body tell me what it needed to heal.

Now that I had put away all of my guilt for being on this trip, I wanted to concentrate on my training. I did exactly what my teacher asked of me and I booked classes with several teachers and studios. I learned rapidly that my body was still a mess! Each class I went to, I could feel my body struggling with pain. I didn't let on very easily though. I had gotten very good at hiding it, only to pay for it later behind closed doors. Each time after training, the pain was

Clarity

shooting up my body and the nerve pain would come back with a vengeance. This was a big alarm for me, since I had just enrolled in a year-long program. I was nervous about being able to sustain the program in this amount of pain. However, I found something interesting, the pain I felt after a yoga session didn't stay for long. The environment of the island and the low stress from the trip somehow allowed me to rest and rebalance quicker than back home.

After trying various classes and journaling about each one, I felt very confident that I picked the right style. One of the last classes I did was with a woman who lived at the base of the mountains. She actually taught Viniyoga™. After taking her relaxing, gentle moving yoga class, I felt like a million bucks. It was an amazing experience sitting next to these enormous mountains, smelling the incense she burned, and listening to the group chant words of healing and positive affirmations. My body was soaking it all up and it was singing and happy. It was the style of yoga that I needed, and fate had happened to present me with exactly the style that I needed to heal. I was beyond excited that things were starting to finally fit together. I knew in my heart that I was on the right path.

Once we returned from Hawaii, my eye was actually still very stable. When we returned, I expected things to get rapidly worse again since the last trip resulted in an immediate appointment with Dr. Stewart. So, I was shocked that my eye seemed to be holding steady. My appointment was still a few weeks away, so Dr. Khan and I started to get to work fast with NAET again. I was handling all of the treatments pretty well. It was tiring at times, trying to allow my body to relearn the correct pathways for the energy to flow. But, I stuck with it to really prove to Dr. Stewart that this worked.

On the day of my appointment, I saw Dr. Khan first. We reviewed my progress and we used muscle testing to see how my eye was doing. The answers were coming back that my eye had made some major jumps in the healing process. Since my eye had seemed to be improving quite quickly, Dr. Khan suggested that I discuss my options again with Dr. Stewart. I was hoping he would allow me to wait on an injection if he saw an improvement too. This was a huge moment for me. I had to be prepared to stand up to Dr. Stewart, trust my heart, and make an educated decision for myself once I saw the scan. I knew he would most likely recommend another injection, but I was hoping he would ultimately let me decide how to move forward with the situation.

May 21, 2018, my whole family and I sat in the waiting room with my binder of past scans in hand. I was so nervous that my legs wouldn't stop trembling. My juvenile eye switching test gave me comfort in knowing my eye was doing really well. The questions started to flood me as we sat and waited to be called back, *Was this the appointment that will change my fate forever? Am I going to need an injection? Will I know if I'm making the right decision?* The questions kept circling my head until the nurse called me back. After going through all the routine checks, I was led back to take the image of my eye. I studied the tech's micro expressions for any hint of bad news. I didn't see any, and my stomach started to swirl with excitement. With my fingers crossed, I headed back to the waiting to wait for my copy of the eye scan. It seemed like forever, but finally the tech slowly walked the paper out to me. It was like a slow-motion video as her sloth like moves formed a half smile. My excitement flew high. I finally looked at the paper after she handed it to me and

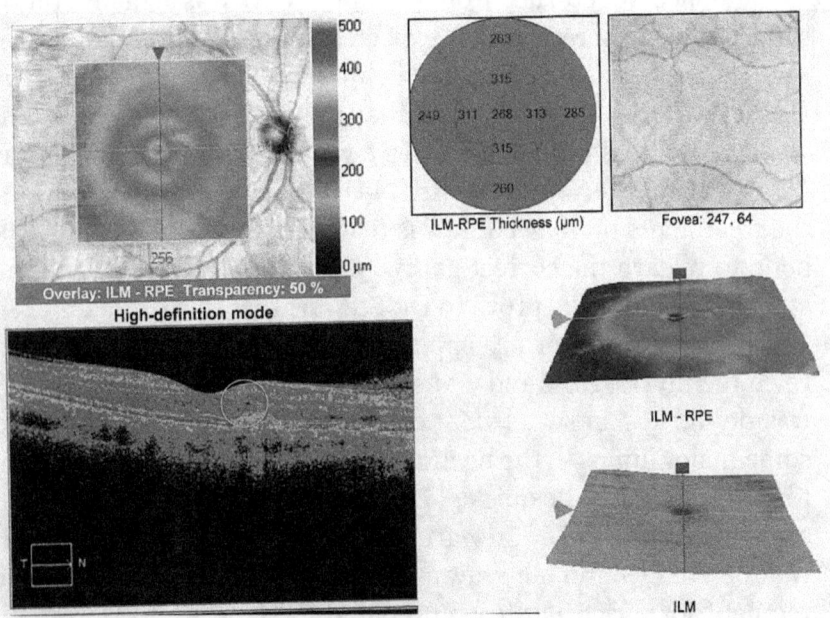

(Photo Caption: OTC Scan taken on 5/21/18 shows the fluid is disappearing.)

Clarity

I noticed the spot was hardly there. I immediately started crying. This was exactly what I needed to see. I was thrilled! "I knew it, I knew it!" I kept saying to my smiling family who shared the same joy as I did.

Now was the big test. What would the doctor say? We sat across from Dr. Stewart; he studied the scan, looked into my eyes with a lighted scope, and said, "Well, your eye looks much better. You've even pushed your appointments apart to six weeks, so the progress I'm seeing looks good. However, there is still fluid in your eye, so the recommended treatment would be to still have an injection." With a pit in my stomach I nervously spoke up, "I think I'm going to decline the injection. I want to see how my body does without it and, since it's not bad right now, I'd like to give my body a chance to heal it." I looked at him with worry and, honestly, Superwoman was standing by ready to argue with him.

As he opened his mouth to speak, I held my breath. Here it was, the moment of truth. Had I just reached a turning point or was I going to get a huge rejection notice? The words finally came out, "I think that's a great idea." Shocked, I stared at him. "Really?!" I shot back. I wasn't expecting that at all! He continued, "Yeah, I think you're incredibly in tune with your body and whatever you're doing right now seems to be working. I think it's a good idea and if you need to come in, I'll make sure we can squeeze you in somewhere. But yeah, let's see what happens. We'll see you back anywhere from four to six weeks." The tears suddenly just started pouring out of my eyes as I shook his hand goodbye. This was beyond exciting! I had worked so hard visualizing all of this playing out, and it really happened! I replayed the words he said to me over and over again in my head. This was the first milestone in my success and it made me feel like I was flying above the clouds!

Now that I had just leaped over my first obstacle, I had to keep a steady pace. To do that, I worked with Dr. Khan as much as possible. We had gotten through all of the foods, chemicals, and environmental issues. Now, we were starting on the big, heartache parts: the events, people, and emotions. This part was extremely touchy because I had to sift through the entire big trauma events in my life. Sometimes, the event that we would be working on made me feel sad or caused physical pain. Only because that is exactly how I felt in the moment of the event. Even though I felt moments of relief from the trauma, I welcomed all of the symptoms as I knew it was progress. I stayed the course because this was my path to fully healing.

  I also worked very closely with my regular eye doctors over the next few weeks to watch and see if the black hole in my eye changed at all. What I found extremely interesting was as I did NAET treatments regarding the events and emotions; the hole would react and also became bigger. I was nervous I would go backwards, but I wanted to see what would happen when my body finished clearing an event. Time would only tell, and I had to do everything I could to keep my body relaxed and steady in the healing progress.

  My yoga training couldn't have started at a more perfect time. Skipping my last injection was exciting, but it also brought a sense of panic. Constantly, I was checking my vision with my juvenile eye switching test and watching how stressed I got. This sense of unease didn't help my nerves to try my first yoga class. I was curious about how my teachers would handle my pain and issues. To my surprise they were gentle, easy going, yet watchful and patient with me. That was a breath of fresh air after getting harped on in some of the other yoga classes I'd taken in Hawaii.

  The hardest part of my training, though, was having to vocalize what caused my pain in my back. I had gotten so used to hiding it, that having to talk about it was uncomfortable for me. I still struggled with not wanting to show weakness, but I knew in this environment I had to learn and I had to ask questions in order to heal my body. At one point, one of the teachers, who happened to be a neurosurgeon, came over to me and asked me to go into child's pose again. He said to me, "I don't know what's going on with the right side of your spine. This is perplexing me. Does your back hurt when you go into this posture?" I said, "Sometimes," as I pointed to my right side and hip area. "Every once in a while, it grips, but it's more the muscles that are pulling. I don't feel it in my spine." He looked at me confused and said, "Umm, we'll have to watch that as you continue on."

The comment made my heart sink. I was so sick of people telling me there was something wrong. I pushed away the tears and continued on. I knew at this point that my right side/back pain was actually coming from my liver and my muscles around it were inflamed. I didn't know how to explain that to the neurosurgeon. I figured he would look at me funny so I didn't elaborate more than I did. I was reminded again on what NAET had taught me; that the liver channel was blocked from all of the allergies I formed from the traumas, and that line of energy blockage was exactly where the pain was coming from.

I tried to stay strong in knowing this and I pushed forward the best I could in class. I knew time was going to be the only thing that I needed at this point. I needed time to learn yoga and to practice the breathing techniques to control my stress and anxiety, I needed time to work with Dr. Khan, I needed time to clear out my trauma, and I needed time for my body to relearn how to heal again. I knew it would come, but it all had to start with loving myself, which meant giving my body the tools it needed to feel good, and to be dedicated to taking that time to heal. At this point, it was all about feeling good, finding happy, and staying positive. My body would correct itself as long as I gave it all the good tools I possibly could.

WHAT I DID AND WHAT YOU CAN DO: ACTION STEPS 25-28

➤ Step 25 - Practice Yoga:

Yoga is an approach in which one can heal the body or slowly learn to gain strength in the body. My suggestion would be to pick a style of yoga that focuses on healing the body in a therapeutic approach, like Viniyoga™, rather than a fast, vigorous style. Learning to relax while doing your yoga practice will allow you to become more connected to that voice you hear within. Sometimes, it can be difficult to sift through all of the thoughts you have going on each day; doing a practice will help re-center your thoughts and keep you on a healing path without all the clutter of stressful ideas.

The other very important aspect to your yoga practice is understanding breath. The idea behind this is the body can live without other senses, but if breath is taken away, the body will fail rather quickly. In our busy lives, we're constantly flooded with difficult situations, which, in turn, cause our bodies to change our natural way of breathing. Let's take, for example, a person who's in a fast-paced, stressful job or a mom who has lots to juggle in her household. Both examples are people in circumstances who are constantly tapping into their sympathetic nervous system, causing the body to eventually start to break down because they're accessing their fight or flight response all day long. Learning to practice yoga daily will help the body start to remember what it feels like to tap into the parasympathetic nervous system, our calm relaxing natural state, and will start to rejuvenate the body.

    A person can go through the movements all day long, but when attached to the concentrated practice of breath, that's where the real healing begins. Our bodies need to be cared for and looked after as the years go on. Life is rather difficult. Some people will have more difficulties than others, but most people struggle with different obstacles in life that trigger a negative emotional response. Yoga is a practice that doesn't take the difficult obstacles away, but helps the body prepare for them. None of us can do any good in the world if we're stressed out and chaotic all the time.

    Yoga, through breath and proper movement, overall help the body and mind to overcome the obstacles in front of us without breaking down the body to get through the difficult time. The movements and the concentration on the breath overall help a person notice habits that are negatively affecting them and, with knowledge, comes change to rewrite the physical response the body is making. My recommendation would be to look up Gary Kraftsow, or, if you're struggling with your eye, you may want to look up eye yoga. There are some helpful exercises that can improve the muscles behind the eye to aid in healing. I've provided some excellent yoga practices on my website at www.nikkiengels.com/yoga

> **Step 26 - Travel:**

    At some point in your healing progress, you're going to feel like spreading your wings a bit and enjoying life to the fullest. That will look very different for each person. However, my recommendation is to get out of your house and your town, and pick another location of the world to visit. Maybe this is some place that you've always dreamt of going, or maybe you have a big adventurous side and you randomly pick a place on the map. Whatever it is, do it! Life is short and your condition can be the motivation you need to do the things you never thought you'd be able to do. Will it be scary? Yes, probably for some people it will be, but the reward of a new place will be worth it. When you spread your wings and let go a little bit, you're going to realize what you're truly happy about.

You'll also learn to be grateful for the little things in life and to be grateful for the experience itself. At least for me, I realized that my eye had pushed me to try new things, and experience more out of the fear that I would never be able to see things again. In return, I was extremely grateful for the push, because it changed my perception of my surroundings and myself. Travel does take you out of your comfort zone, but you'll feel more powerful and determined to handle your situation once you start living your life to the fullest.

➢ **Step 27 - Love Yourself:**

Loving yourself is one of those phrases that you probably have heard at some time in your life. Most of us hear it and roll our eyes, thinking, *Yeah, yeah, what does that even mean?* This is a hard idea to think about, especially when you're going through the rough grieving stages in the beginning. Sometimes, when your body stops working the way it should, you'll fill yourself with negative thoughts, and you might feel frustrated with the event itself.

It's important to do things for yourself that encourage healing rather than doing things that are destructive to your body. For example, picking up a bad habit like excessive drinking, isn't going to heal your situation, but picking up a healing book or doing yoga will point you in the right direction to heal. Really use your inner voice to help you navigate through this. Only do the things that make you feel whole, alive, and centered in your way of thinking. If an event or an opportunity doesn't sit well with you or causes you stress, then sit back and reevaluate it. Maybe there's a reason you don't want to take that opportunity, or maybe it does excite you and you're scared. If it's the latter, you might want to take the jump and push yourself.

This is a time to really sit back and ask yourself what you want for your life. What makes you happy? The answer to that question is most likely what you need to do to love yourself. Loving yourself is all about listening to that inner voice/your heart, taking the time to relax, setting your sights on a goal that you would love to accomplish, and going out there and doing it. Loving yourself is simply doing what makes you the happiest.

> **Step 28 - Take Safe Chances:**

You may reach a point in your healing when you'll have to listen to your inner voice and go against what you're being advised. Now, I have to say for legal reasons, I don't recommend going against your doctor's recommendations. However, I'm saying that you need to make sure you don't lose your voice and your intuition throughout your healing. For me, I was able to safely decide to hold off on treatment, but I knew I could be seen right away if problems arose. This gave me the wiggle room I needed to see if my eye would heal without the injection. If you're in a more serious condition, be sure to take all of your doctor's recommendations into account and safely decide what you feel is right.

Intuition is such an important part of healing. Your subconscious knows what it needs to heal the condition you have. Often, for myself, I ignored that intuition and later had regrets about it. As you're healing your condition, ask your doctors lots of questions and see if you can find a little wiggle room to make good, educated decisions about aspects of your healing. For me, I was able to space out my injections. I stayed within the guidelines, but I pushed them out as far as I could. Once I proved to Dr. Stewart that I was doing great with that, he was able to give me more wiggle room. So overall, work with your doctors, don't forget you have a voice and an opinion, and take the wiggle room they give you to heal your condition the way you feel is best for you. You'll most likely be surprised how fast little decisions add up to your main goal of being completely healed. As my husband always says, "Little things add up to be big things."

Clarity

** YOUR TO-DO LIST **

25. PRACTICE YOGA EVERY DAY.
26. PICK A LOCATION, GO VISIT IT, REFLECT IN YOUR JOURNAL ON HOW YOU FEEL
27. TAKE THE TIME YOU NEED FOR YOURSELF, GUILT FREE.
28. FIND WIGGLE ROOM WITH YOUR DOCTOR TO SET SMALL GOALS.

Chapter 9:
Taking My Life Back With NAET

Over the next five weeks, I kept working very closely with Dr. Khan. We were deep into using the NAET protocol to go back through the events of my life that were contributing factors of my eye misbehaving. Some of the most interesting events were the most recent traumas I had gone through. The stressful time in my life of rebuilding our home, taking care of our sick son, and also running the coffee shop and our martial arts school became the forefront of my healing. These events were intertwined in so many different ways.

To someone watching from afar, they would have never known how to untangle the mess. But my body seemed to understand which order I had to clear them in. As soon as I would be done clearing a section, my body would start throwing warning signals for the next knot I had to untangle. Strangely, I would experience phantom pain that I had back at that time, or memories of that time would keep popping up in my head. Once I started to see the clear signs of the next piece of the puzzle, it was easy for me to show up in Dr. Khan's office and explain to him what I thought we had to do next. It always surprised him a bit on how I would walk in with the answer. We often chuckled about the process and my long written lists of things I knew were connected to the next piece of the puzzle.

At this point, I had gotten really good at intuitively knowing what came next in my healing process. I knew going into this that it would be long, since only I knew how much I shoved down the

Clarity

emotional trauma. Having to, piece by piece, dig it up and get rid of it for good was a liberating feeling. My body actually started to respond so well to releasing the emotional baggage I collected, that my nerve pain was completely gone and I was able to eat most of the foods that I was previously having trouble with. Now, that also meant things I had previously cleared would pop up again, but it was connected in a new way to the event I was currently working on. It all depended on the invisible knot of emotions I was working on. For example, while clearing the house fire, I would feel like I had been crying all night, and my nerve pain would spike from the amount of stress my body had been under at that time. I would also feel about 20 minutes or less of sadness, and some of the foods connected were eggs and wheat. If I ate the food while I was clearing this section, my stomach would react in a similar fashion as it did when the event actually took place. As my body started to push the negative energy through my system, I would get a sense of relief. It was an interesting process to be able to physically and emotionally feel when the event was traveling through my system.

Now, to some people whom I've talked to, they don't feel much of anything while they're clearing. Others, like myself, feel a whole host of different emotions and physical responses. Everyone is a bit different in how they absorb and feel emotions, and each person clears these negative energies out in different ways as well. At times, this can be a long process; however, remember that the body didn't break down overnight. It might have felt like it, but looking back, multiple things added up to the body breaking down.

Knowing this about myself, I was able to stay the course and I kept working hard to push as much negative energy out. The hard work paid off when I went back to see Dr. Stewart five weeks after I told him I'd like to skip the injection. He was thrilled about the progress and said, "Your eye is holding steady. It looks relatively the same as it did five weeks ago. It's been about 11 weeks since your last injection, there is a little fluid in the eye, but it looks like it's draining out just as fast as it's coming in. And your inflammation hasn't changed either. I can do an injection today if you'd like, since there is fluid in the eye, but I think you're doing fine without it. What would you like to do?" I, of course, declined the injection, and booked my next appointment for six weeks out.

I was absolutely thrilled! This process was working! I could feel the stress of life literally evaporating from my body every time I did a NAET treatment, yoga practice, or just spending time reading a good book. I finally was making progress and knew it was largely due to NAET and all the other necessary changes I made previously that contributed to the progress. I always said to my family that the stress I felt for so long was wearing me down. It took a catastrophic event in my body, to get me to make the changes I needed and get off the hamster wheel.

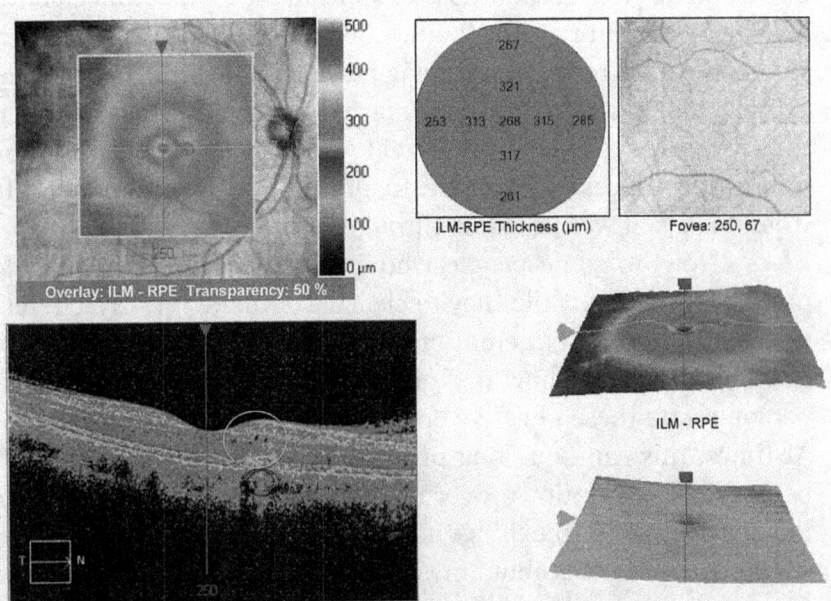

(Photo Caption: OTC Scan taken on 6/27/18. The image shows the fluid is staying steady without medication after 11 weeks since an injection.)

Things only kept getting better from here on out. I followed up with Dr. Stewart again over the next few months and kept pushing my appointments out without an injection. Finally, on September 26th, 2018 he allowed me to push my appointment out to six months with the comment of saying "Your eye is rock solid!" I had hit another amazing milestone in my healing progress. Feeling extremely grateful, I kept up using all the tools that I had

Clarity

accumulated and, one-by-one, started stripping the hurt, frustration, and sadness away. I started to wake up earlier, feel alive again, and my pain was completely gone. That is, if I wasn't clearing something at the time. Food also was so much easier for me to enjoy now. I was able to eat foods like eggs again without feeling absolutely exhausted. I was starting to get my life back. To make things even better, my attitude had completely changed for the better. My husband said that I wasn't getting bogged down by things that use to be stressful to me. I was able to let go of stressful events and people without feeling a nasty tug-of-war on my heart. Life just seemed more colorful, bright, and full of possibilities without all the negative trauma filling me up and blocking the free-spirited person that I was deep down.

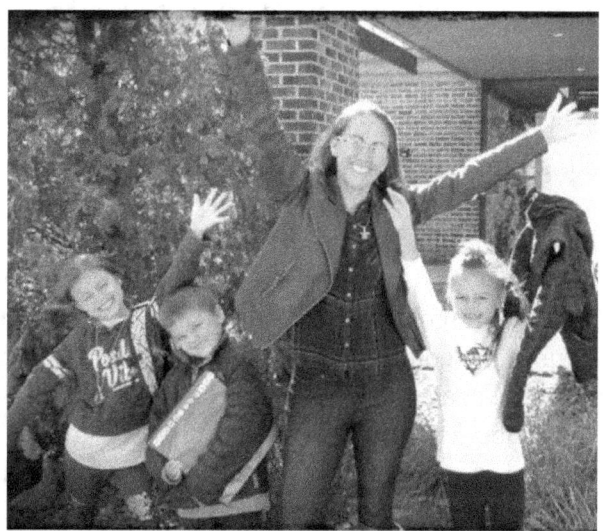

(Photo Caption: Photo taken by Gary Engels on 9/26/18. Nikki stands with her kids in celebration outside of Dr. Stewart's clinic after he cleared her for six months. Her son holds his mom's health binder with pride.)

The more I used my tools, the better things got. I kept visualizing every day my doctors being completely taken aback by my success. I wanted them to say the words that I was totally healed. That I had absolutely done it, and that they didn't have an answer for it. Since my doctors didn't understand Eastern medicine, I wanted to show them and hopefully stick the question in their mind of, "How did she do that?" I hoped that I could change their perspectives from being doom and gloom, to anything is possible.

The time had finally come. It was March 13, 2019, six months from the last time I had seen Dr. Stewart and about 11 months since my last injection. I was extremely excited for the appointment. Yet habits of nerves still sat there wondering what he was going to say when he saw my OTC scans. I kept working hard on visualizing my success throughout the prior weeks. Dr. Khan and I also gave my body a few weeks' break from the NAET treatments to let my body settle down from all the hard work I was putting it through. I still saw Dr. Khan three times a week but only to work on keeping my neck muscles loose. This seemed to help keep my body relaxed and healing as well. I also had been consistent on taking enough vitamin A to support my eye, and I continued eating extremely well to give my body the other proper nutrients it needed. I was doing everything I possibly could to get to the result of hearing Dr. Stewart say the words I so desperately needed to hear.

Walking into the waiting room, I was jittery, yet confident. My family was excited for me as they sat in the chairs with huge smiles on their faces. I had just finished all of the preliminary tests before I could see Dr. Stewart. The nurse proudly walked across the waiting room to hand me the scan. She had a smile on her face from ear to ear. I knew she couldn't say anything about the scan results, but I could also tell she couldn't hold back her excitement for me. I looked at the image and the hole was completely gone. My chest filled with flutters of excitement as I tried to hold back the tears. I had done it, but I still didn't know what the doctor was going to say.

Finally, we were called back to see him. He walked in with a large smile on his face, shook our hands like old friends and said, "Let's take a peek." He leaned me back in the chair, quickly shined a bright light in my eye to look at the retina, tipped my chair back up and then said, "At this point you've shown you can get past six months plus some without an injection. Currently, the fluid is gone. There's really no reason for you to come here just to have us take a picture of your eye every so often. I'm going to discharge you from the clinic today. You don't have to come back here anymore unless a problem arises. But, your chances of that happening at this point

Clarity

are extremely low." I think I about fell out of the chair. I was discharged!? What?! I didn't expect him to say that at all. I assumed I would be cleared for another six months or a year. To be discharged was beyond my scope of thinking, but I was thrilled! I literally had done it! I had gone from needing these injections for the rest of my life, to two and a half years later completely healing it! The tears flooded my face as my family jumped from their seats to hug me! The doctor kept his composure under his big smile, said goodbye to us, and walked out of the room.

We slowly gathered our things after we poured our emotions out in the room. My family had walked out into the hallway before me and I was the last to leave the room. As I walked out, I passed a young man who was about the same age as me, maybe a little younger. He was struggling to see out of one of his eyes. His emotions were pulsating from him and I could feel and see that he was struggling with what appeared to be the start of his healing journey.

As we passed each other, my heart skipped a beat for a moment. That was me two years ago. I so wished I would have been able to talk to him and encourage him as he walked back to see the same specialist I did. I didn't know what his condition was, but considering this was a clinic of retinal specialist, I could only guess that it was going to be something major.

At that moment, I decided to write this book. My hope is that whoever reads this story can follow some or all of the tips I've laid out to help themselves heal. If I could have talked to that man, I would have told him, "The healing power is within you, you just have to find it." To all of my readers who need a little encouragement, You've got this! You can do this and I believe in you!

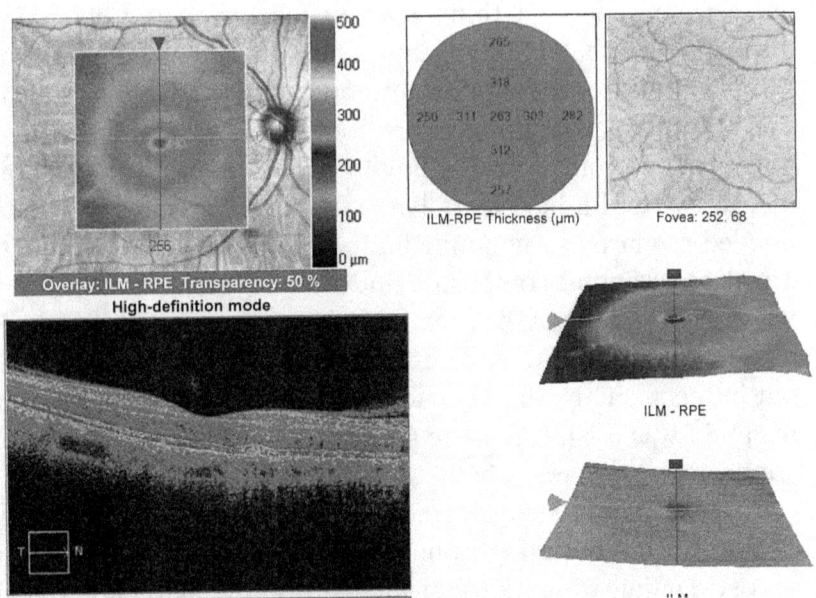

(Photo Caption: OTC Scan taken on 3/13/19 shows the retina has healed and the fluid is gone. The numbers also reflect the changes.)

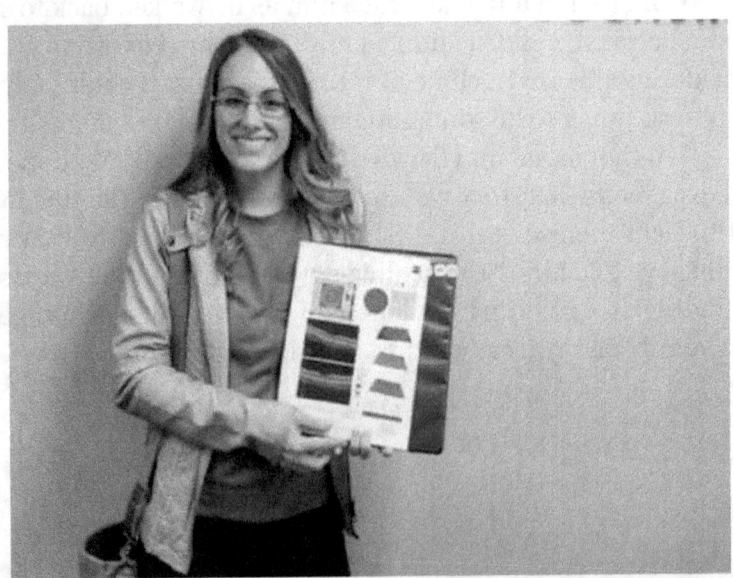

(Photo Caption: Standing at the appointment desk, I took this picture to mark the end of this journey with my successful scan in my hands and my trusted binder of information.)

Clarity

WHAT I DID AND WHAT YOU CAN DO: ACTION STEP 29

> **Step 29 - Learn NAET:**

This protocol was a turning point in my healing journey. With the combination of the other things I did, I was able to find out what was happening in my body when all of my other doctors didn't have the answers. NAET was again developed by Devi S. Nambudripad, M.D., D.C., L.Ac., Ph.D. (Acu.). She also wrote a book called *Say Good-Bye to Illness*. Within her writing, she goes into a deeper understanding of what an allergy is. I think this is important to understand so that you can see how you may have formed allergies to different things in your life that you would never think of.

Dr. Devi states that allergies are caused from *"Energy blockages and imbalances caused in the body's energy circulation by various factors:*

a. Heredity (inherited from parents, grandparents, uncles, aunts, etc.)

b. Toxins from various sources. Toxins are produced from the interaction between the person and the unsuitable energies of foods, drinks, chemicals, pesticides, environmental factors, bacteria, fungus, virus, mercury, MSG, etc.

c. Lowering the immune system due to extra stress put on the person's body, causing the body to become weak and over-reactive towards other energies. The commonly seen stressors are: physical injuries, accidents, surgery, serious illness, and emotional injuries.

d. Deficiency and malabsorption disorders, producing abnormal enzymes leading to abnormal functions in the body (poop digestion, causing anaphylaxis, hormonal disorders, abnormal thyroid functions, etc.)

e. Overexposure to toxic substances (chemicals, attic insulation material, pesticides, allergic foods and drinks, food additives, food colorings, extreme cold, heat, etc.,) over a period of time.

f. Emotional factors and traumas creating sudden stops in the energy functions leading to chronic blockages in the energy circulation (sudden sadness, joy, trauma, or painful memories of various incidents from past and present, causing the unusual immune response).

g. Toxins caused from physical exertion like vigorous exercise, running, playing sports, etc. Toxins (produced in the body from: bacterial or viral infections; molds, yeast, fungus or parasitic infestation; constant contacts with certain irritants like mercury, lead, copper, chemicals, etc.).

h. Radiation (excessive exposure of television, sun, radioactive materials, etc.)."

Dr. Nambudripad also discusses that these allergies can be cleared from your system by using her NAET protocol. She defines her protocol as *"a non-invasive, drug free, natural solution to eliminate allergies of all types and intensities (mild sensitivity, to severe hypersensitivity reactions, to severe anaphylactic reactions (successfully treated peanuts, penicillin, aspirins, mushroom, shellfish, etc., and the patients can use them in their everyday life now without any adverse reactions) and allergy-related disorders (some of the examples: common colds to severe infections; learning disabilities to autism and ADHD; anger and clinical depression to schizophrenias and various other mental disorders; mild join pains, arthritis of different types and intensities, small cysts and skin eruptions to tumors and growths, angina pains, high blood pressure to strokes, all arising from allergies to food, environmental toxins, chemical toxins, and emotional stressors) and often with lasting results."*[15]

We all know that stress defines us. It literally tells us how we're feeling, how we act, how we think.... All of it. So, why is it so hard for our society to understand that our emotions are in the driver's seat of how we function as a human being? Our emotions, with their own personalities, are literally doing the steering of how we react to different events. Let's say that you find yourself in a situation and suddenly feel anxious, which most of us have from

Clarity

time to time. But where did that emotion come from. Why did it just come out of the blue and hit you in the chest like a lightning bolt. As you dart your eyes around and wonder what on earth caused this sudden feeling of breathlessness, you realize something is familiar, but you can't quite put your finger on it. This is the time when you need to step back. Ask yourself, what in this current moment is really the cause of the anxiety. Is it the time of day? Is it the colors in the sky? Is it possibly the people you're with and the things they're saying? Try to tune into the inner you and ask yourself what it is. No one can hear what you're thinking. So, take a moment, breathe, and ask yourself the hard questions. When you start to tap into those triggered responses, start asking yourself if it's possible that you're allergic to some of it. Chances are you do have an allergy to something if it's causing a negative feeling or reaction in your body of some sort.

My suggestion would be to look up a practitioner near you who does the NAET protocol. You can find more information at www.nikkiengels.com/NAET. The steps I've listed throughout the book aren't completely necessary for you to have success with NAET But, in my opinion, if you do these steps, you'll have a much more solid approach to learning about yourself throughout the NAET protocol. Remember, it took you a long time to develop your situation, and it will take some time and some hard work to get out of it. Stick with it, keep fighting and moving forward, and you'll find the solution you need to heal your condition.

Chapter 10:
Make Growing Your Goal

Currently, my eye is doing great. My condition is still at the status of healed and I am now working on dissolving the scar tissue in my right eye from the original burst blood vessel. I am still diligently working with Dr. Khan with the NAET protocol to rebalance my energy to keep progressing forward. At this point, my eye doctors have stated that dissolving the scar tissue would be nearly impossible. I'm a firm believer that it can be done, and I have learned to smile at the challenge. Although I can now wear my contacts from time to time at home and in Hawaii, I'm still working hard to fix the prism that developed because of my situation.

My theory is if I can dissolve the scar tissue completely, then the prism will be gone since my eyes won't have to work so hard anymore. Since I know how well NAET and a healthy lifestyle worked to heal the bleeding, I'm confident to say the other goals will be achieved in the very near future. My other symptoms: food allergies, nerve pain, and my back/side pain, have completely gone away. Every once in a while, if I do the NAET protocol and clear an allergy from those difficult years, I'll feel some of those symptoms come back. However, it's a lot easier to understand and to accept when you know it's a short moment of discomfort.

When I'm not clearing, I live in a very peaceful state of relaxed thoughts and emotions and without the physical pain. My relationships have blossomed, and my family life has gotten so much happier and free now that we don't have to worry about all the food restrictions any more. To top it all off, since starting this journey, everyone in my family has benefited with being happier and overall healthier. My daughters are thriving at school and they no longer need reading glasses because their eyes have improved as well. My son's breathing is tremendously better, and we haven't had to worry about giving him medications for his lungs for the past two years. It truly has been a blessing to watch how my trauma has positively impacted us all in a positive way. It was a hard journey, but I'm proud of whom I've become from it.

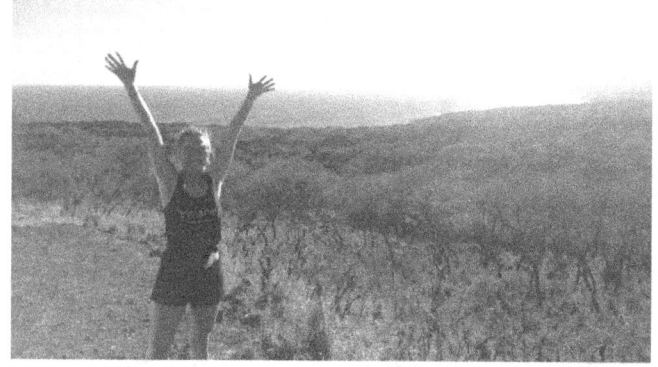

(Photo Caption: After getting our great news, we went to Hawaii to celebrate! This is me after a long and scary adventure. I did it!)

I want to extend to you that no matter what you're going through, you can do this, and there can be a purpose to your heartache. You just have to change your perspective, find your answers, heal your body, and keep pushing for a healthier and happier you, both physically and mentally. I know you can do this! Find your voice, live your life to the fullest, and be grateful for all the positive things in your life. When you focus on the positive, positive will come your way.

WHAT I DID AND WHAT YOU CAN DO: ACTION STEP 30

> **Step 30 - Celebrate:**

You did it! You healed yourself! Now it's time to celebrate you and your success! Decide how you'd like to do that and make it a priority! Congratulations on all your hard work!

Resources Page

Please also look into joining my website at www.nikkiengels.com for more resources.

Website Resources:
1. https://www.retinalphysician.com/issues/2017/october-2017/treatment-of-focal-vs-diffuse-diabetic-macular-ede
2. https://studyres.com/doc/7188243/avastin%C2%AE--bevacizumab--intravitreal-injection
3. https://draxe.com/health/eye-health/macular-degeneration-symptoms/
4. https://draxe.com/5-gut-types-quiz/
5. https://draxe.com/health/gut-health/candida-symptoms/
6. https://draxe.com/health/gut-health/leaky-gut-diet-treatment/
7. https://s3.amazonaws.com/draxe/Programs/HealingLeakyGut/Deliverables/Immune+Gut+Plan+-+Healing+Leaky+Gut+by+Dr.+Josh+Axe.pdf
8. https://s3.amazonaws.com/draxe/Programs/HealingLeakyGut/Deliverables/Candida+Gut+Plan+-+Healing+Leaky+Gut+by+Dr.+Josh+Axe.pdf
9. https://www.health.harvard.edu/blog/leaky-gut-what-is-it-and-what-does-it-mean-for-you-2017092212451
10. https://healgrief.org/stages-of-grief/?gclid=CjwKCAjw7anqBRALEiwAgvGgm7r7xHXP-FhxKMuiRR_DKagzu9GtzOZppYm5-U_nXT7zuVGtmqFoiBoCoTIQAvD_BwE
11. https://www.byodo-in.com/
12. https://www.byodo-in.com/bon-sho.htm
13. https://www.youtube.com/watch?time_continue=8&v=tdlAcHh68wE
14. *The Hidden Messages in Water* by Masaru Emoto.
15. *Say Good-Bye to Illness*. Nambudripad's Allergy Elimination Techniques. A Revolutionary Treatment for Allergies and Allergy-Related Conditions. - Devi S. Nambudripad, M.D., D.C., L.Ac., Ph.D. (Acu.) Pgs. XXXIX and XLI

About the Author

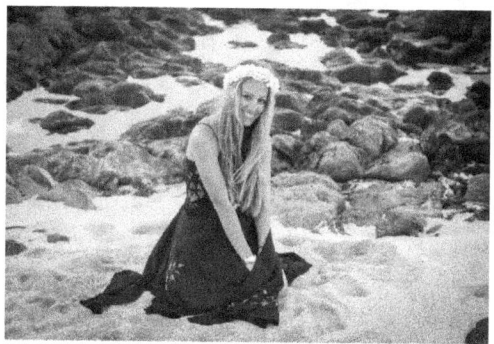

Nikki Engels is a wife and mother of three beautiful children. She has dedicated her career of 14 years to teaching women how to stay active and healthy through her teachings in her women's fitness classes and kickboxing classes. She has taken her passion to help others one step further by becoming certified in Viniyoga™ and writing about her healing transformation that took place from 2016 to 2019. Nikki is dedicated to teaching others that they too can heal conditions similar to hers through various natural ideals.

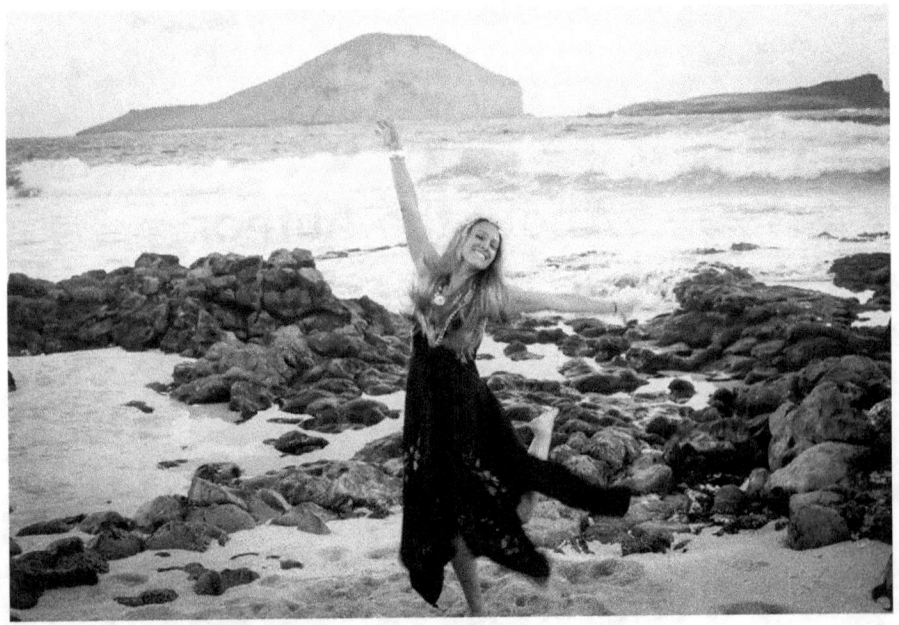

Thank You for Reading My Book!

I really appreciate all of your feedback, and I love hearing what you have to say. Please share your story and how this book has impacted your life.

Please leave me an honest review on Amazon letting me know what you thought of the book.

Thank you so much!

Nikki Engels

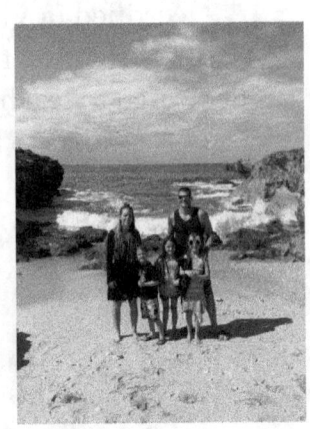

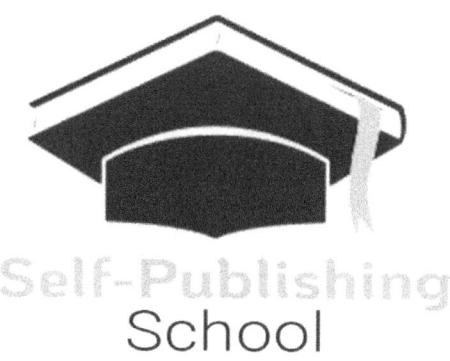

NOW IT'S YOUR TURN

Discover the EXACT 3-step blueprint you need to become a bestselling author in 3 months.

Self-Publishing School helped me, and now I want them to help you with this FREE WEBINAR!

Even if you're busy, bad at writing, or don't know where to start, you CAN write a bestseller and build your best life.

With tools and experience across a variety of niches and professions, Self-Publishing School is the only resource you need to take your book to the finish line!

**DON'T WAIT
Watch this FREE WEBINAR now, and Say "YES" to becoming a bestseller:**
http://nikkiengels.com/sps (all lowercase)
Click on "Join Our Free Training"

www.ingramcontent.com/pod-product-compliance
Lightning Source LLC
Chambersburg PA
CBHW051402290426
44108CB00015B/2121